THE WORLD
OF
PERFUME

© Copyright Paris 1995
This edition published in North America in 1996
by KNICKERBOCKER PRESS
276 Fifth Avenue Suite 206
New York, New York 10001

designer: Jacqueline Leymarie
editor: Marina Zmak
translation: Mark Howarth
English language edition: Cathy Muscat

ISBN: 1-57715-004-X
Printed in Spain

Fabienne PAVIA

THE WORLD
OF
PERFUME

*Photographs
Matthieu Prier*

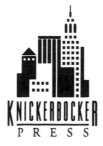

KNICKERBOCKER
PRESS

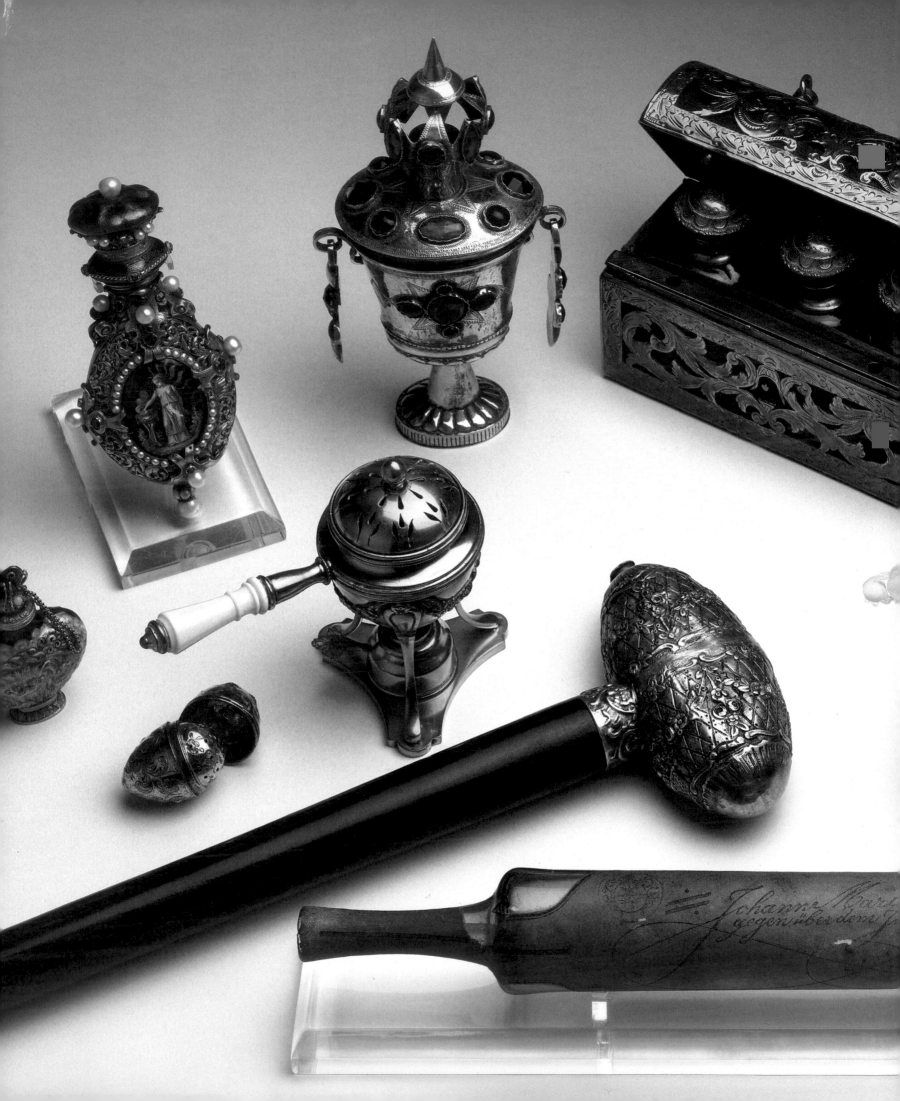

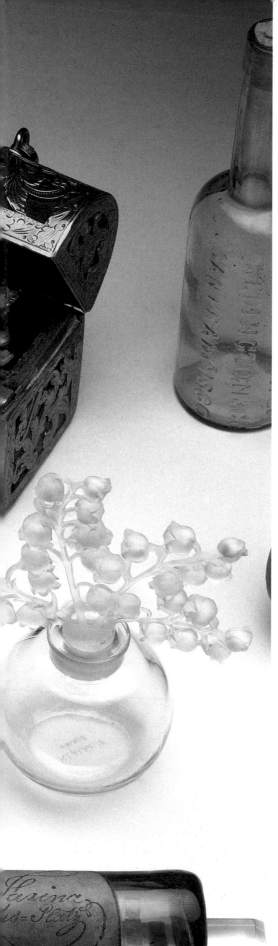

CONTENTS

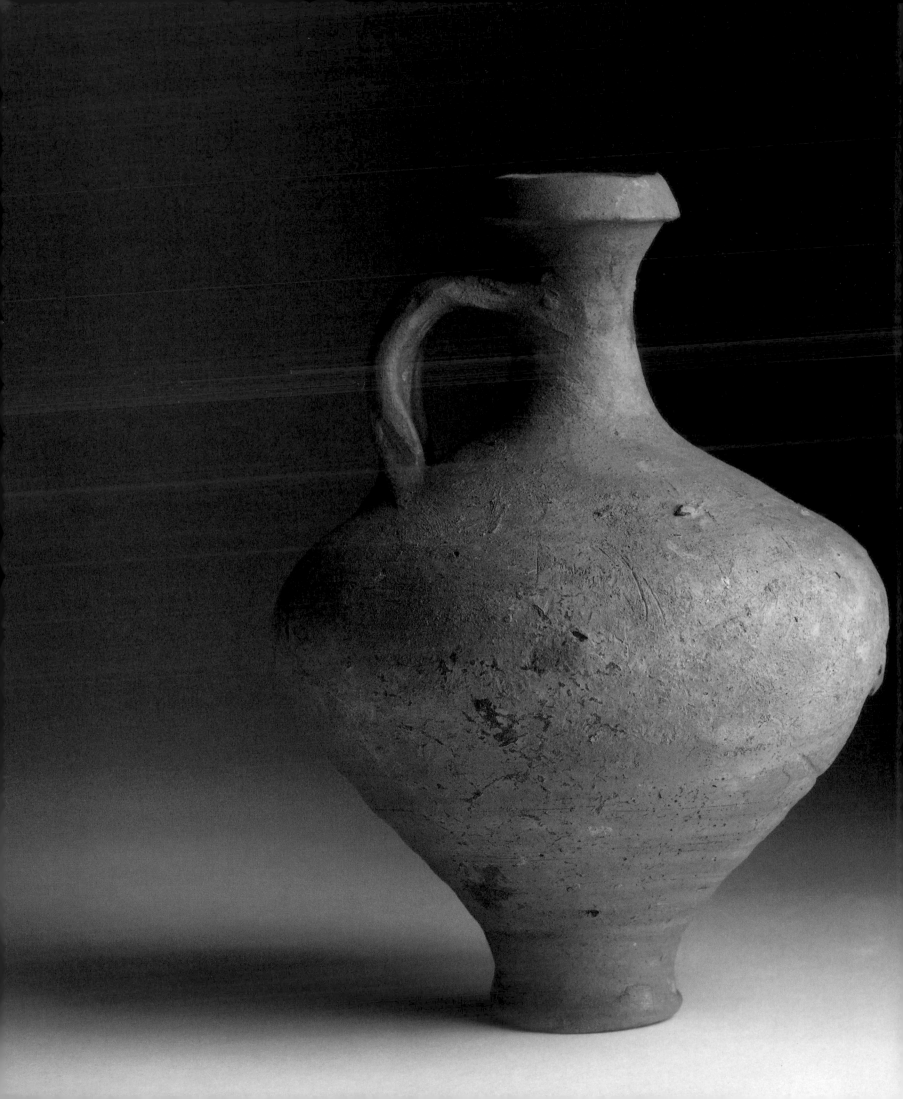

THE HISTORY OF PERFUME

The history of perfume is intimately linked with the development of mankind. Since prehistoric times, man has improved the flavor of food by burning aromatic oils and woods. The Ancient Egyptians honored their gods with incense and ointments and fragrant oils became an essential part of both religious ceremony and a woman's beauty regime. The Greeks returned from their voyages with new fragrances, while in Ancient Rome perfumes were believed to possess medicinal properties. The use of perfume declined in Europe as a result of the barbarian invasions, but new developments in the art of perfumery were made in the Islamic world. Through the invention of the still and their perfection of distillation techniques, the Arabs and Persians became the undisputed masters in the use of aromatics.

It was not until the twelfth century that the Christian world rediscovered the attractions of perfume, both because it symbolized elegance and for reasons of hygiene – it was worn to ward off plague and noxious odors. The sixteenth century saw the merging of the glove and perfume-making trades, as the contemporary fashion was for perfumed gloves. Though the medieval upper classes washed regularly, the practice was abandoned during the two centuries after the Renaissance as a result of the Council of Trent. Perfume sales therefore increased due to the need to disguise unpleasant smells.

In the seventeenth century, civet and musk were the fashion, while a preference for sweet, floral and fruity fragrances took over during the Enlightenment. Seduction was the keynote of the eighteenth century. There was a profusion of new fragrances and bottles, and perfume was even added to the ashes on Ash Wednesday. Further advances in chemistry in the nineteenth century enabled the artificial reproduction of naturally occurring fragrances as well as the creation of new ones. Perfume manufacture on an industrial scale was born and Grasse, France established itself at the center of this flourishing trade.

Luxury and progress being hallmarks of the twentieth century, perfume has continued to retain its cachet, entering the privileged world of art, as well as the ruthless arena of commerce.

Roman terracotta jug for scented oils, c. 300 AD.

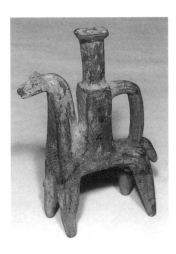

Left: *Perfume was first used by the Egyptians as part of their religious rituals. Note the "incense arm" which was used for fumigations in honor of the gods.*
Right: *Grey earthenware kohl vase in the shape of a horse, Urartu, Asia Minor, 9th-8th century BC.*

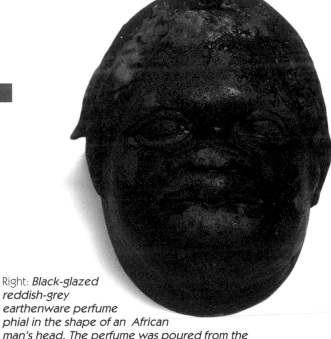

Right: *Black-glazed reddish-grey earthenware perfume phial in the shape of an African man's head. The perfume was poured from the hole in the middle of the scalp.*

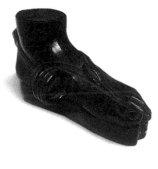

Above: *Black-glazed Alexandrian ceramic guttus in the shape of a foot wearing a Roman sandal. It could be carried using the ring on its side. Like the African head above, it comes from the necropolis of Arg el-Ghazouani, Kerkuane, late 4th-early 3rd century BC.*
Right: *Bronze oil lamp, Rome, 3rd-4th century AD.*

PERFUME IN ANTIQUITY

ANCIENT EGYPT

Although perfume in the modern sense of an alcohol-based solution did not exist in Ancient Egypt, fragrant substances played an essential role in this great civilization. There were two principal methods of use at this time: the burning of incense and the application of balms and ointments. The practice of fumigation consisted simply in placing wood, spice, fruit or resin over a heat source and allowing the perfume to dissipate into the air. This custom soon became a regular practice in the temples, where basic raw and untreated substances were gradually replaced by increasingly complex blends. Evidence of this has been found in the hieroglyphics discovered at Edfou and Philae which have provided us with valuable information on the evolution of perfume. By deciphering the ancient script, detailed recipes for early fragrant blends were revealed. Thus, the ingredients for the well-known incense kyphi – myrrh, lentisk, juniper, fenugreek seed, pistachio and chufa – were first ground and sifted. The resultant powder was blended first with wine and then with a boiled down liquid based on conifer resin and honey. The Egyptians used two devices for burning incense: a metal charcoal burner and an "incense arm." This was a kind of sleeve carved out of wood or cast in bronze, with an open hand at one end supporting a small cup which contained the incense.

Ointments and perfumed oils were applied to the skin for either cosmetic or medicinal purposes. As distillation, and therefore pure alcohol, was unknown at the time, fatty substances such as vegetable oil and animal fat were used to absorb the fragrance of a flower or resin. Colorants and preservatives were subsequently added to this base. Ointments were stored either in pots or vases which were usually made of alabaster. Small earthenware, stone or ceramic bottles, generally in the shape of an animal, were also used. Bottles made of glass appeared later in the form of multi-colored jugs, amphoras, vases and goblets.

During the Old and Middle Kingdoms, perfumes were reserved exclusively for religious rituals such as cleansing ceremonies, the annointing of the dead and the worship of the Gods. They eventually came into secular use during the festivals of the New Kingdom (1580-1085 BC), each of which called for a specific fragrance, even though they were still prepared by priests. Egyptian women also used perfumed creams and oils as toiletries or cosmetics and as preludes to love-making.

GREECE

Following in the footsteps of the Egyptians, the Greeks developed a wider range of perfumed products and extolled their virtues for both religious and everyday use. It was considered fashionable to coat the body in oils and creams when bathing and before and after meals, for reasons of hygiene as well as pleasure. The Greeks believed perfume to be a gift of the Gods. The bodies of the dead were perfumed before burial along with their personal effects, which always included a scent bottle. The spherical aryballos made the direct application of creams onto the skin possible. They were produced in Corinth along with alabaster vases and lecythi, one-handled vessels decorated in the Athenian style. From the sixth century BC onwards, bottles made in Rhodes took on more original shapes: sandalled feet, busts of the Gods, animals, mermaids and so on.

ROME

Drawing on influences from the Orient and Greece, the Romans were quick to invest perfume with great prestige, even though Julius Caesar suppressed the use of exotic fragrances. The use of perfumes in funerals and religious ceremonies, as well as in daily life, became more widespread, thanks largely to the extension of trade routes as far as India, Africa and Arabia. As the trade of perfume-seller was often associated with that of doctor or apothecary, the Romans regarded perfume as having medicinal properties. One of their great innovations was the use of glass containers (balsam jars, lachrymatories, phials and ampullae) and they developed the technique of glass-blowing invented in Syria in the first century BC.

THE ISLAMIC WORLD

The spread of Christianity led to a decline in the use of perfume in the western world, both in daily life, where it was considered frivolous, and in religious ritual, where the custom of burying personal belongings along with the deceased disappeared. By contrast, the Arabs kept it alive through the flourishing spice trade, the invention of the still and improvements in techniques of distillation. The gardens of the Alhambra palace, in the southern Spanish town of Granada, provide ample evidence of their sophistication and the role that fragrances played in people's everyday lives. After all, Mohammed asserted that what he loved most in the world was "women, children and perfume." Europe had to wait until the Crusades and the intervention of a few Venetian crusaders, who were driven more by a quest for earthly pleasures than for divine faith, to discover the use of soap and rediscover the appeal of perfume.

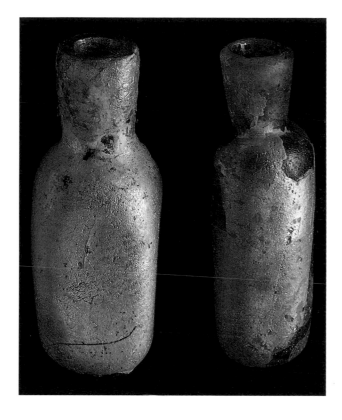

Small perfume bottles in iridescent glass, Iran, 8th-10th century AD. Perfumes and spices had been widely used in Iran since time immemorial. At one stage, the caliph of Baghdad would regularly order thirty thousand bottles of rose water per year.

9

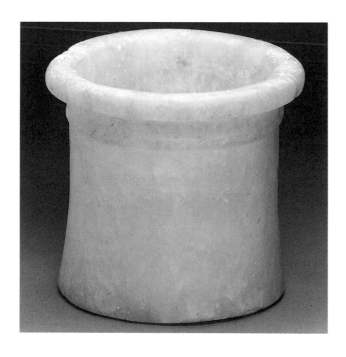

Cylindrical ointment jar, Egypt, 1st Dynasty, c. 3000 BC.

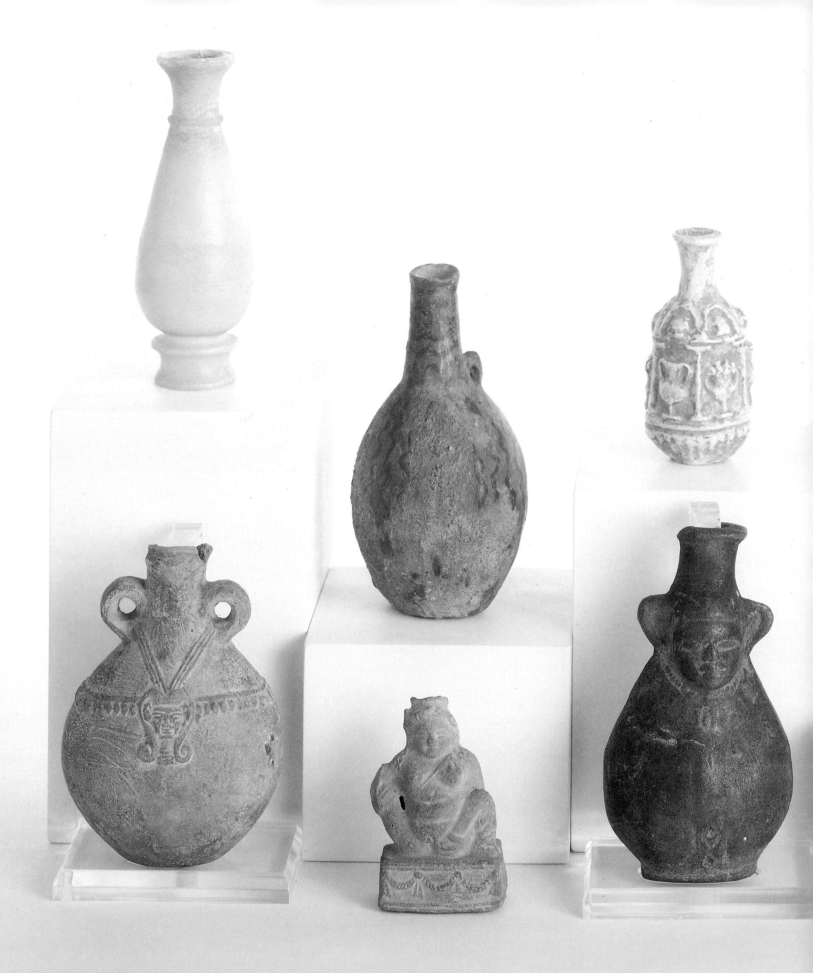

10

Top, left to right:
Alabaster vase used for religious ceremonies, Egypt, c. 1350 BC.
Terracotta balsam pot, Cyprus, 2000-1600 BC.
Opaque white moulded glass balsam pot, decorated in the Roman style, 100 BC-100 AD.

Bottom, left to right:
Marbled stone ointment pot, Egypt, c. 1500 BC.
Terracotta pot for balsam or holy oil, depicting a woman in an erotic pose, Egypt, 300-200 BC.
Black clay pot for holy oil depicting the goddess Hathor, Egypt, c. 400 BC.

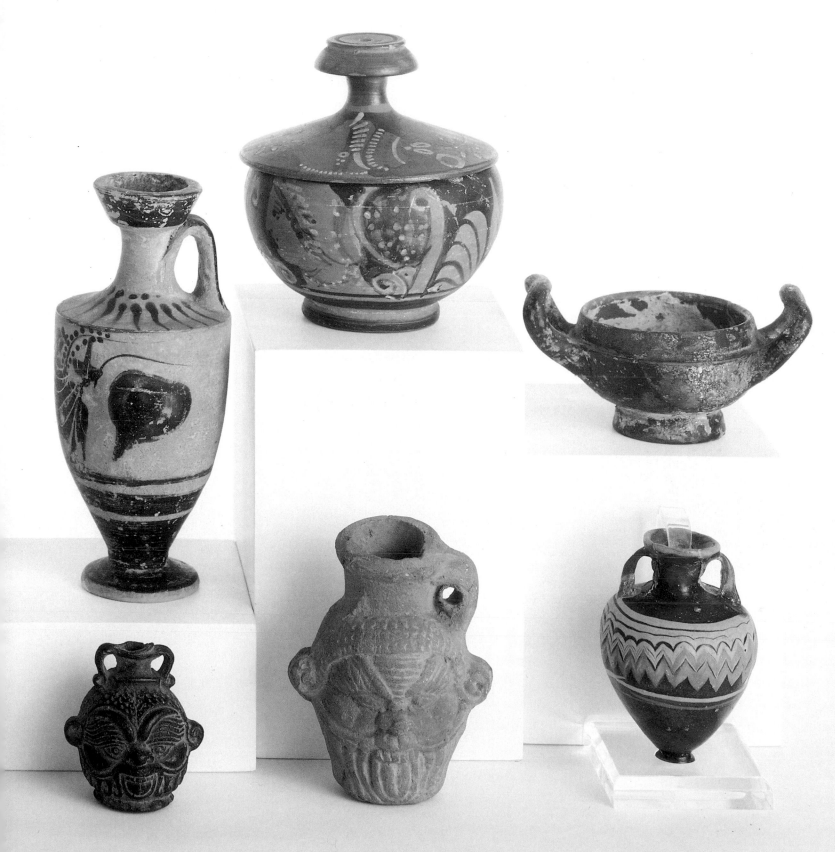

Top, left to right:
Terracotta lecythus painted in the Athenian style. Its red interior denotes that it contained perfumed oils intended for secular use, c. 500 BC.
Ointment pot, Greece, c. 400 BC.
Grecian terracotta incense burner, southern Italy, 400-300 BC.

Bottom, left to right:
Clay balsam pot depicting the head of a god with two faces, late Ptolemaic Egypt, c. 100 BC.
Moulded terracotta balsam jug. Each side depicts the face of the god Bes, the great protector. Ptolemaic Egypt, 300-100 BC.
Small Phoenician amphora in ultramarine glass with yellow and turquoise painted motifs, c. 700 BC.

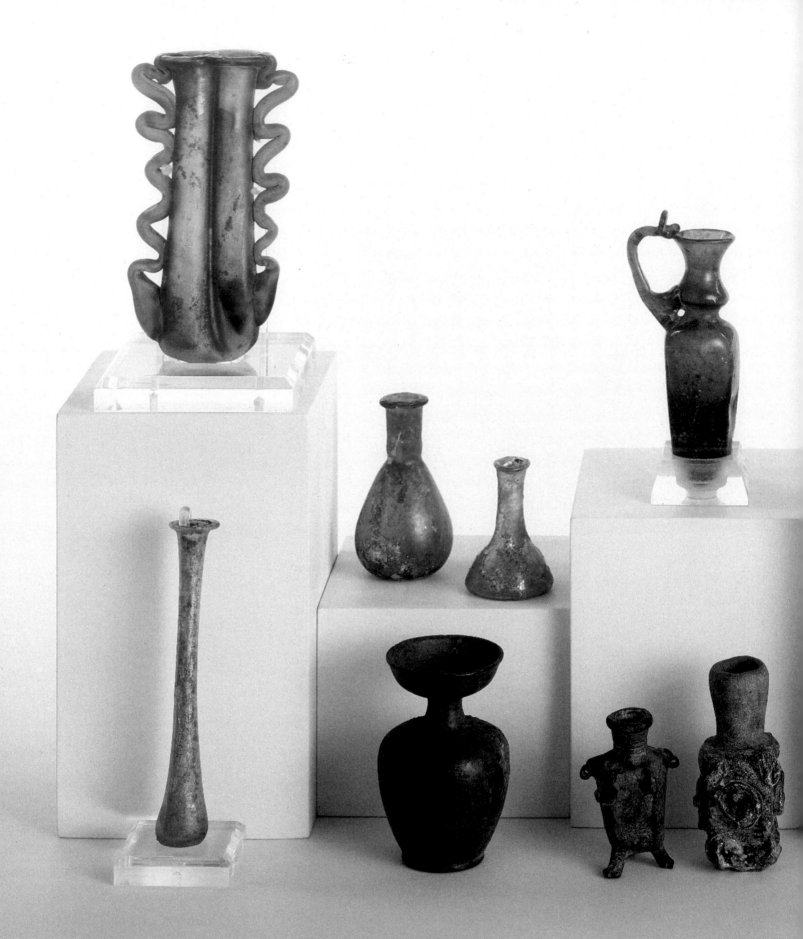

12

Top, left to right:
*Twin-vessel balsam pot in iridescent blue-green glass with filament
decoration at the sides, eastern Mediterranean, 2nd-4th century AD.
Small Roman bottles for scented oil, one in iridescent cobalt blue
glass, 2nd-3rd century AD.
Glass ointment jar, north-eastern Iran, 10th century AD.*

Bottom, left to right:
*Roman glass phial, produced during the reign of Julius Caesar.
Roman bronze balsam pot, 1st-2nd century AD.
Bronze bottle, Iran, 12th century AD.
Glass bottle, northern Iran, 4th-6th century AD.*

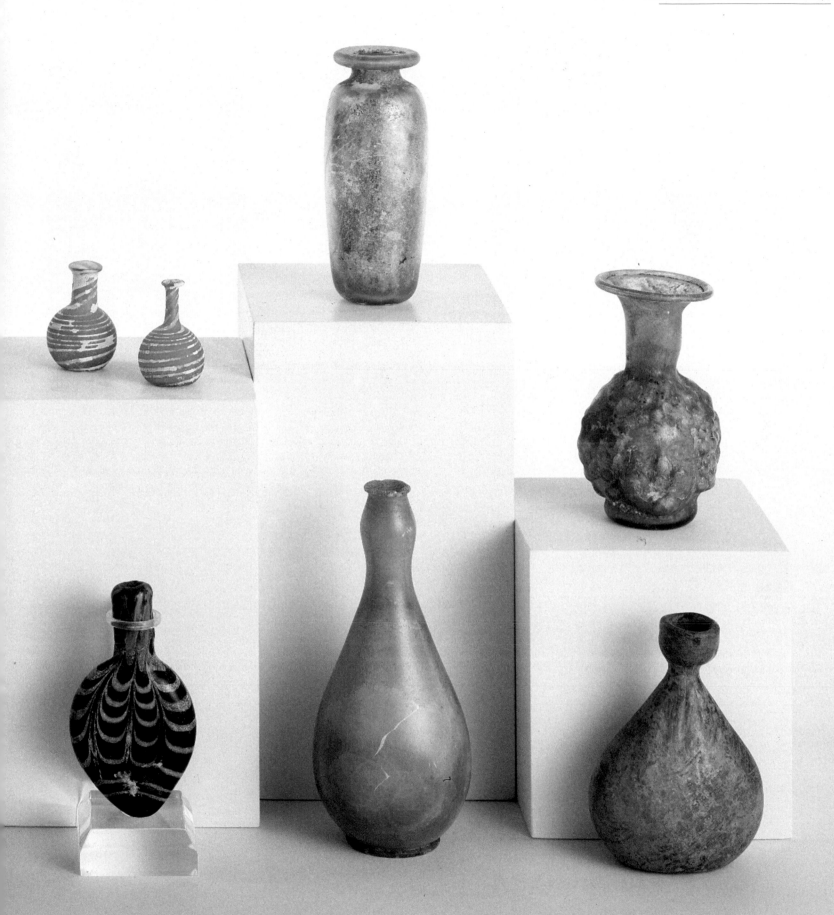

Top, left to right:
*Small balsam jars, one in blue glass with white spiral decoration,
Iran, 2nd-3rd century AD.
Green glass jar, Rome, 200-100 BC.
Roman balsam jar in greenish yellow blown glass, depicting the
heads of two women with luxuriant hair, 1st century AD.*

Bottom, left to right:
*Islamic enamelled glass bottle, 6th-9th century AD.
Alabaster vase, Middle East.
Glass bottle, Iran, second half of the 3rd century AD.*

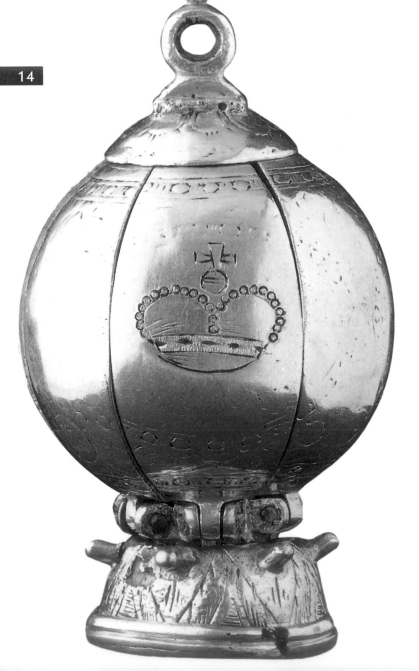

Round silver gilt pomander engraved with a crown. The silver mount has an openworked base and contained a fragrant substance. The ring unscrews to open the pomander, which is divided into six segments decorated with delicate engravings of plants. The sliding lid of each compartment bears the name of the scent inside. Germany, 16th century.

FROM THE MEDIEVAL TO THE BAROQUE

The fall of the Roman Empire, barbarian invasions and interminable war plunged the Western world into the Dark Ages and perfume's influence dwindled. It was not until the twelfth century and the development of international trade that this decline was reversed. The establishment of universities in major cities, coupled with a mastery of alchemy and distillation learned from the Arabs, led to increasing knowledge of perfume manufacturing techniques. While frankincense and myrrh remained sacred fragrances, kings, nobles and courtiers discovered the hygienic and seductive properties of perfume. The beauties of the day sprayed their garments and their homes with an aspergillum similar to the device used to sprinkle holy water in religious ceremonies. They would regularly bathe in water perfumed with the essence of flowers and coat their bodies in scented oils just as the Athenians used to do, although with rather more restraint. Contrary to received wisdom, washing and bathing were widely advocated during the Middle Ages. A new container designed to hold musk, ambergris and fragrant oils and resins was invented – the pomander was a metal globe which emitted perfume through its openworked decoration. These fragrances were believed to have therapeutic properties designed to ward off plague and other epidemics, aid digestion, preserve fertility and treat impotence.

As most of the spices coming into Europe from the Orient passed through Venice, the city quickly established itself as the capital of perfumery. Marco Polo returned from his voyages with pepper, nutmeg and cloves. Arab sailors followed the spice route as far as India and Ceylon, where they could trade with Asian merchants who imported spices from China and Malaysia, and brought back cinnamon, ginger, saffron and cardamom. Aniseed, thyme, basil, sage and cumin had already been cultivated in Europe for some time.

The second half of the fourteenth century saw the appearance of liquid perfumes, produced by blending essential oils with alcohol, known as *eaux de senteur* or scents. There is an interesting story attached to the first of these to be created, which was made from rosemary and named after the queen of Hungary. Legend has it that the scent was given to Queen Elizabeth of Hungary by a monk in 1380. She was 70 years old at the time and in a poor state of health, but when she drank the liquor (in those days these preparations were drunk) her health improved. Such were its rejuvenating effects that the king of Poland requested her hand in marriage.

With the discovery of the Americas in the fifteenth century, Venice would lose its pre-eminence. First the Portuguese and then the Spanish expanded the trade in spices, dealing in vanilla, cocoa, tobacco, cinnamon and so forth. In the sixteenth century the Dutch also enjoyed great success in this field: unlike their predecessors, who had confined themselves solely to trading, they supervised production overseas and improved methods of cultivation.

Eaux de senteur increased in number and came in one of two varieties: plain, which was composed of a single fragrance (such as rose, lavender or orange flower), or blended, which partnered flowers and spices with musk and ambergris. In addition to their pharmaceutical potential, these helped to disguise bodily odors. While the Middle Ages was a period that set great store by personal hygiene, things were seen quite differently during the Renaissance, a time when water was suspected of carrying plague and other infections. Glass-blowers employed Venetian techniques to produce phials and ampoules for perfume, and crystal and milky-white glass reminiscent of oriental porcelain also became popular. Pear-shaped bottles, made from both base and precious metals, appeared in large numbers and the pomander became more elaborate, with small compartments like the segments of an orange, each of which could be filled with a different scent.

Perfume enjoyed huge success during the seventeenth century. A great craze for it developed – perhaps in inverse proportion to the contemporary standards of cleanliness – and the faces and wigs at the court of Louis XIV were fragrant with powders and perfumes. In 1656, the guild of glove and perfume-makers was established. For some time, the passion of the upper classes for wearing gloves had been tempered by poor tanning methods, which caused the gloves to leave a nauseating odor on the skin. Strong fragrances were therefore used to perfume them. With the patronage first of Louis XIII and then Louis XIV, the guild of glove-makers took the opportunity to acquire the monopoly of perfume distribution at the expense of apothecaries, distillers, alchemists and chemists. The seventeenth century also saw jasmine, tuberose and rose join the range of materials used in perfume manufacture. The pomander came into more widespread use, remaining in vogue until the end of the eighteenth century, and bottles were produced in ever more varied designs, such as pear-shaped, and made from colored, crystalline transparent glass or opaline. Engraved silver gilt was particularly popular, as were enamelled copper, silver and gold or semiprecious stones. With the baroque period came pouncet boxes and bottle cases with exotic decorations.

15

Gilded bronze perfume-burner with the entwined body of a snake slithering through the burner itself. France, Louis XIV.

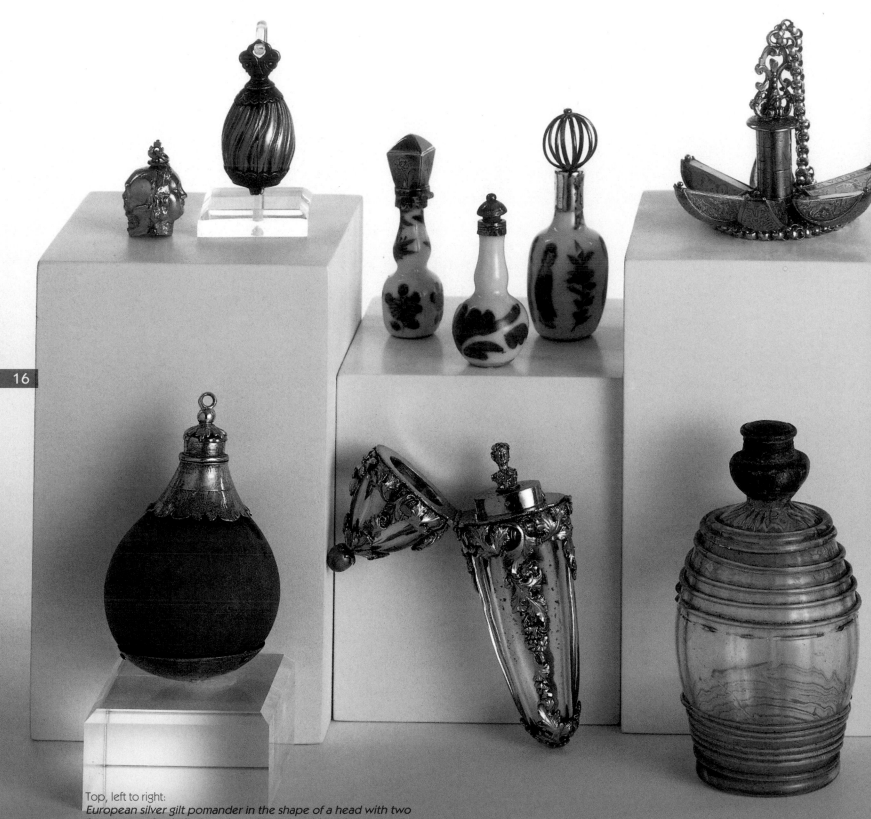

Top, left to right:
European silver gilt pomander in the shape of a head with two faces, one of a skull, the other of a young girl, 16th century.
Silver pomander, Germany, 17th century.
Small porcelain bottles, China, 17th-18th century.
Sumptuously engraved silver gilt pomander. The hook unscrews to open the pomander, which is divided into six segments arranged around a central cylinder, each bearing the name of a fragrance. The sides of each segment are engraved with hunting scenes. When reassembled, they form a sphere. Southern Germany, late 16th century.

Bottom, left to right:
Ebony and silver bottle, Germany, late 17th century.
Crystal bottle with silver gilt mount and lid set with a pearl, France, late 17th century.
Glass bottle, Germany, 17th century.

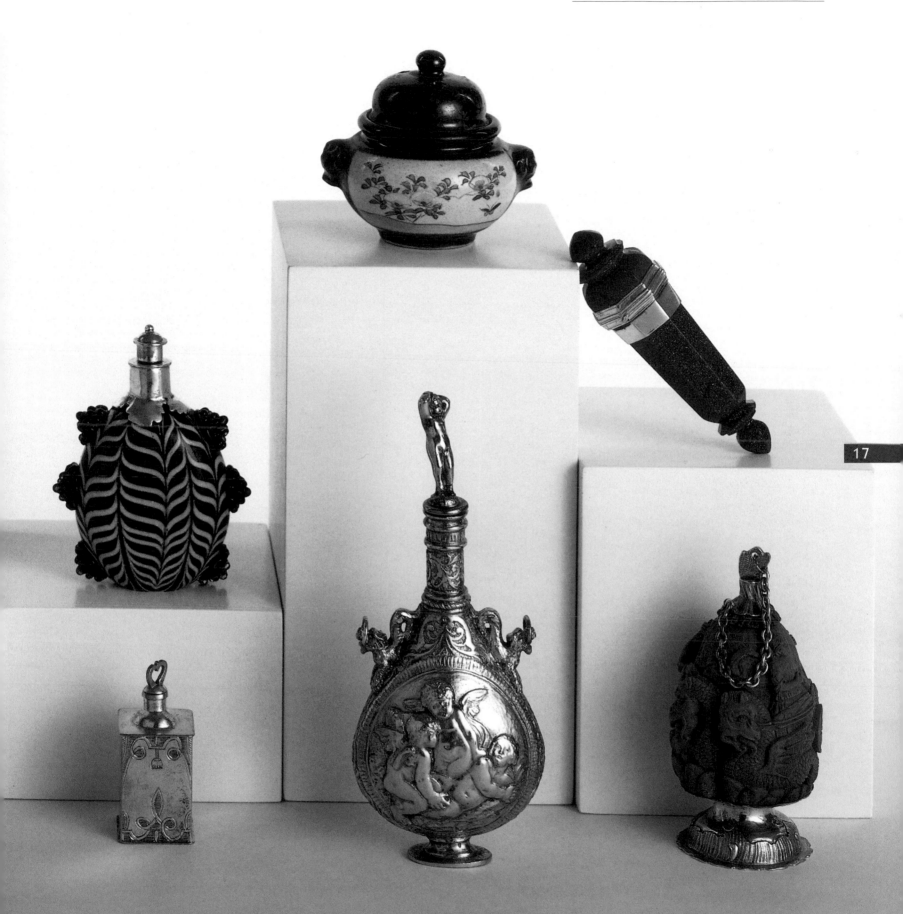

17

Top, left to right:
Glass bottle, Holland, 17th century.
Ceramic pot-pourri jar in the shape of a tureen with an openworked lid, painted with flowers on one side and a domestic interior on the other, China.
German or French carved aventurine bottle with silver mount, late 17th century.

Bottom, left to right:
Silver bottle, Emden, Germany, c. 1680.
Silver gilt bottle produced by the court workshops in Prague, decorated with bas-reliefs copied from paintings by Bartholomeus Spranger and Hans von Aachen, 1580-1600.
Carved coquilla nut bottle with silver mount, Portugal or Spain, 17th century.

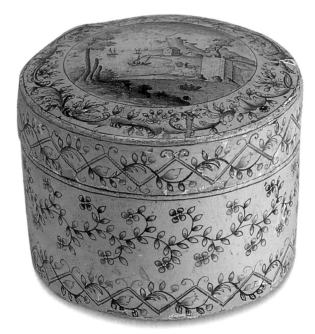

Vanity box with portraits of Marie Antoinette and Louis XVI, France, 18th century.

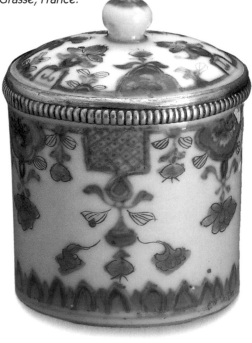

Round bergamot box. These boxes were very popular in the 18th century and were often given as love tokens. Grasse, France.

Porcelain pomade jar, early 18th century.

THE AGE OF ENLIGHTENMENT

In France, the century of the great philosophers and the French Revolution was also the age of perfume. The court of Louis XV was even named "the perfumed court" due to the scents which were applied daily not only to the skin but also to clothing, fans and furniture.

While *eaux de senteur* continued to be widely used, competition appeared in the shape of *vinaigres de toilette* or salts, which were reputed to have unrivalled disinfectant properties. The most famous of them, the "four thieves" *vinaigre*, enjoyed remarkable success in Marseilles during the terrible plague of 1720. Four grave robbers were believed to have been protected from contracting the disease thanks to a concoction of their own invention. Once arrested, the villains' lives were spared in return for giving the authorities the recipe for their miraculous potion, which was immediately posted on every wall in the city. It seems safe to assume that the effectiveness of this *vinaigre* lay in its ability to repel insects, the main carriers of the epidemic.

The eighteenth century saw a revolutionary advance in perfumery with the invention of eau de Cologne. This refreshing blend of rosemary, neroli (orange flower), bergamot and lemon was used in a multitude of different ways: diluted in bath water (bathing became an increasingly regular practice in the eighteenth century); mixed with wine; eaten on a sugar lump; as a mouthwash, an enema or an ingredient for a poultice; injected directly... the list is endless. The controversies surrounding its invention could fill a book of their own and inspired a bitter rivalry between the Feminis and Farina families. The least convincing theory names the Farina family from Emilia in northern Italy as the inventors of a perfume which was originally to have been called eau de Bologna. The more generally accepted version begins in the fourteenth century at the convent of Santa Maria Novella in Florence, where the nuns made *aqua reginae*. Such was its success that in the seventeenth century a certain Giovanni Paolo Feminis went as far as seducing the convent's mother superior in order to make her disclose the recipe. Establishing himself as an apothecary in Cologne, he lost no time in reproducing and marketing his discovery, which he first named "Eau Admirable" before settling on "Eau de Cologne." Feminis later summoned from Italy a nephew, Gian Maria Farina, who expanded his uncle's business considerably in the years up to 1766. However, this was not the end of the story. Other Farinas, claiming to have invented eau de Cologne, soon appeared and by 1865 there were no less than thirty-nine shops in Cologne bearing the name. Nevertheless, one Jean-Marie Farina (nobody knows whether the name was real or assumed) distinguished himself with the perfumery business which he established in Paris in 1806. The quality of his perfume, coupled with great business acumen, set the seal on his reputation – Napoleon, one of the greatest consumers of the fragrance, ate it on a sugar lump.

Another version of events dates back to 1792 and the wedding, at the head office of Mülhens Bank in Cologne, of the banker's son Wilhelm. One of the guests, a monk, gave the young couple a manuscript containing the recipe for a scent with medicinal properties called *aqua mirabilis*, which the groom subsequently marketed under the name of "4711, the true eau de Cologne." (4711 was the number of his house, as designated by Napoleon's army). Two hundred years later, his descendant Ferdinand Mülhens still sells the fragrance.

The variety of eighteenth-century perfume containers was as wide as that of the fragrances and their uses. Sponges soaked in scented *vinaigres de toilette* were kept in gilded metal vinaigrettes. Liquid perfumes came in beautiful Louis XIV-style pear-shaped bottles. Glass became increasingly popular, particularly in France with the opening of the Baccarat factory in 1765 and the concentration of the Saint-Louis glassworks on the production of perfume bottles – the fame that their crystal soon acquired remains to this day. Jewelers produced bottles in engraved gold and silver, studded with jasper or quartz. The style of decoration broke with the baroque and drew inspiration from more contemporary themes such as chinoiserie and Rousseau's cherished return to nature. Chinese decoration adorned Chantilly porcelain bottles, whereas the Saint-Cloud factory was famous for its gilding and Sèvres for its pear-shaped bottles. However, porcelain was above all the preserve of the Germans, the Austrians and the English. The Chelsea factory specialized in figures, mainly human but also animals and fruit, the heads of which formed the stoppers while Wedgwood bottles came in the characteristic blue and white designs. In Germany, the Meissen factory was the first in Europe to use hard paste in its porcelain. Rococo designs, oriental motifs, flowers, fruit and battles were the favored decorations. As with Chelsea, there were also figures, the most popular being characters from the *Commedia dell'Arte*.

The eighteenth century was also the age of the *nécessaire,* a small container for bottles of perfume. As well as the little funnel used to fill the bottles, these *nécessaires* were designed to contain a variety of other 'indispensable' items such as pencils, toothbrushes and even "tongue-scrapers" and small sticks to clean the ears.

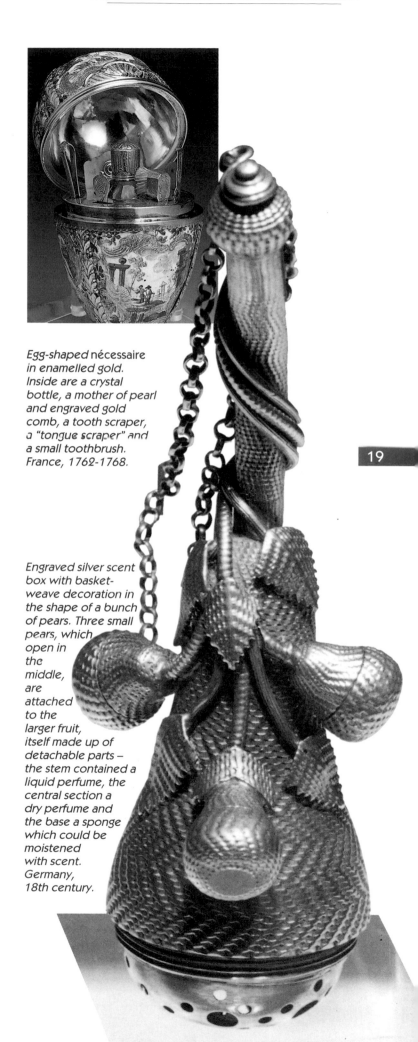

Egg-shaped nécessaire *in enamelled gold. Inside are a crystal bottle, a mother of pearl and engraved gold comb, a tooth scraper, a "tongue scraper" and a small toothbrush. France, 1762-1768.*

Engraved silver scent box with basket-weave decoration in the shape of a bunch of pears. Three small pears, which open in the middle, are attached to the larger fruit, itself made up of detachable parts – the stem contained a liquid perfume, the central section a dry perfume and the base a sponge which could be moistened with scent. Germany, 18th century.

19

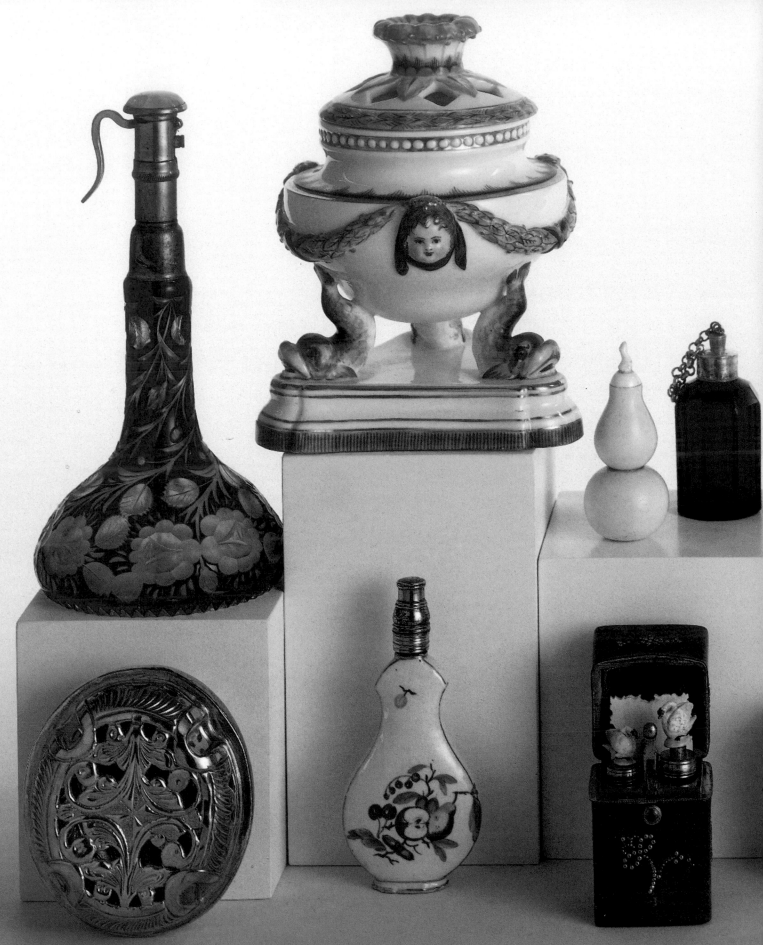

Top, left to right:
Glass bottle with brass fittings, Bohemia, 19th century.
Porcelain pot-pourri jar with dolphin feet, decorated with laurel
garlands and three reliefs of a young girl's face, Copenhagen,
Denmark, 1780-1790.
Ivory bottle, Japan, 18th century.
Ruby-colored glass bottle with silver stopper, Germany,
18th century.

Bottom, left to right:
Silver vinaigrette, Germany, 18th century.
Porcelain bottle with painted fruit decoration and silver gilt
screw-top, Frankenthal, Germany, 1762-1794.
Nécessaire covered in green shagreen leather containing two glass
bottles with swan-shaped porcelain stoppers (Chelsea or Derby).
The box, typical of the 18th century, also contains a writing kit
with an ivory pad-holder, a pencil, etc. England, c. 1770.

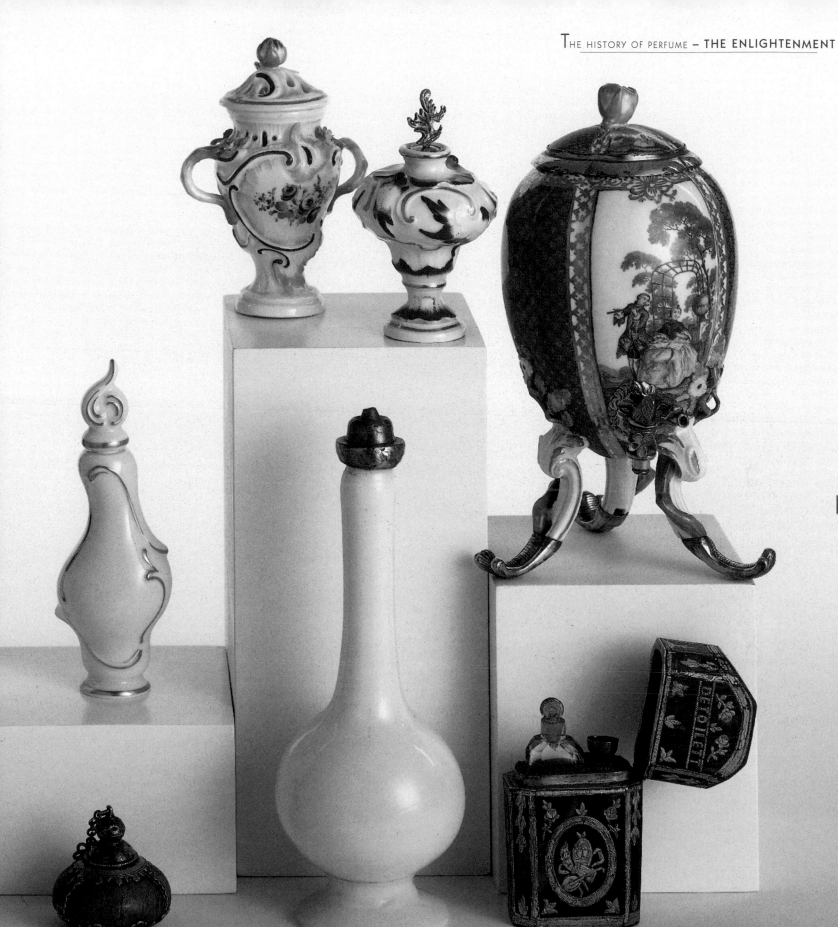

Top, left to right:
Hoechst porcelain bottle, from a design of 1758.
Porcelain pot-pourri jar, Meissen, Germany, c. 1760.
Porcelain bottle, Vienna, c. 1770-1780.
Porcelain perfume fountain, Meissen, Germany, c. 1745.

Bottom, left to right:
Bottle carved from a real chestnut, silver mount, Germany, 1792.
Opalescent glass atomizer with pewter stopper, Germany,
18th century.
Nécessaire containing a glass bottle with silver stopper, Germany
or Austria, early 19th century.

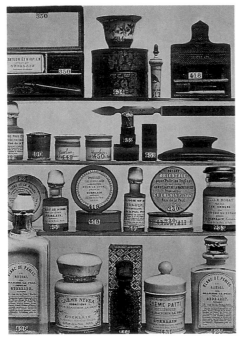

Perfume did not escape 19th-century industrialization. Alchemy gave way to chemistry and new fragrances were created.

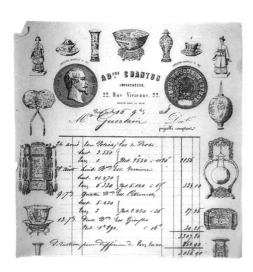

1828 saw the famous name of Guerlain enter the enclave of perfume-making. As well as perfumes, this illustrious company also sold powders, oils and creams.

Invoice from a raw materials producer addressed to Guerlain, 1858. The use of high quality materials was one of the company's founding principles.

THE DAWN OF MODERN PERFUMERY

As with industry and the arts, perfume was to undergo profound change in the nineteenth century. Changing tastes and the development of modern chemistry laid the foundations of perfumery as we know it today.

The French Revolution had in no way diminished the taste for perfume – there was even a fragrance called "Parfum à la Guillotine." Under the post-revolutionary government, people once again dared to express a penchant for luxury goods, including perfume. It became highly fashionable during the Empire as Napoleon and his court were themselves great perfume consumers. Josephine, whose Creole roots had left her with a passion for heady aromas, was even dubbed "Lady Musk." She spent a fortune each year at Lubin and Houbigant, her favorite perfume-makers, and her dressing-room at Malmaison was so drenched with the combined scents of musk, civet, vanilla and ambergris that they still hung in the air seventy years later. The emperor himself had an ambivalent attitude towards perfumes. In fact he hardly liked them at all, at least those which contained artificial fragrances, and found the atmosphere in Josephine's bedroom so stifling that on more than one occasion he was forced to leave. That said, his valet massaged him from head to toe each day with Jean-Marie Farina's eau de Cologne. The perfume-maker had even created a cylindrical bottle for the emperor, which he slipped inside his boots. He would get through as many as sixty a month, for he said that it stimulated his brain. Judging by his correspondence, scents had a similar effect on his love life: "Don't wash, I am on my way and will be with you in a week," he wrote to Josephine.

The Restoration saw a return to more restrained styles of perfume. The vogue was for subtle, floral fragrances rather than animal aromas. Perfumes called *Les Larmes de l'Aurore* and *L'Eau des Belles* were fashionable in the reign of Louis XVIII, while under Charles X *Dame Blanche* or *Troubadour* were worn. Smelling salts, those inseparable companions of languid beauties, were made fashionable by the Romantics. During the Second Empire, the Empress Eugénie revived the taste for heady, patchouli-based perfumes, but this gradually waned in favor of the increasingly subtle fragrances produced by perfume-makers.

Largely due to its jasmine, rose and orange-growing trades, the town of Grasse in Provence soon established itself as the largest production center for raw materials derived from plants. The town had long had indirect links with perfumery through its tanneries and the combined glove and perfume-making industry, which gradually became separate professions once again. The statutes of the perfume-makers of Grasse were passed in 1724, firmly establishing the town's principal industry at around the same time as the introduction of the modern still. The years between about 1770 and 1900 saw the birth of large companies whose names reflect the increasing industrialization of the perfume business: Chiris (1768), L.T. Piver (1774), Lantier (1795), Roure-Bertrand-Dupont (1820), Sozio (1840), Robertet (1850) and Payan-Bertrand (1854).

Paris quickly established itself as the commercial counterpart to Grasse and the world center of perfume. As well as Houbigant, Lubin and L.T. Piver, the name of Jean-Marie Farina was still in existence. Having first been bought by a certain Léonce Collas, the business was subsequently sold to two cousins by marriage, Armand Roger and Charles Gallet.

The house of Roger & Gallet played a pivotal role in the development of modern perfumery with its adventurous fragrances and high-quality soaps (which are still produced today), as well as its remarkably beautiful packaging and labelling. It was at this time that another important name emerged – one which was to found a perfume dynasty. In 1828, a young doctor and chemist by the name of Pierre-François Pascal Guerlain opened a shop on the rue de Rivoli selling his own powders and perfumes. One of them, *Eau de Cologne Impériale*, earned him the honor of Empress Eugénie's royal warrant. His sons Aimé and Gabriel succeeded him, creating their famous perfume *Jicky* at the very end of the century.

However, the most important advance of the nineteenth century, and the one that brought perfumery into the industrial age, came with the emergence of organic chemistry. This allowed scientists to isolate fragrant molecules and reproduce them synthetically. They could thus give free rein to their imagination and create blends of perfume which did not exist in nature. A new profession came into being which was to gain true recognition in the twentieth century and transform perfume into an art form – that of perfume-blender.

The industrialization of bottle manufacture was a gradual process which did not impinge on high-quality craftsmanship. Crystal retained its cachet, the factories of Bohemia, France and Britain being the finest exponents of the technique. The century's most important development in this field was made by the gastronome Brillat-Savarin, with his invention in 1870 of the atomizer.

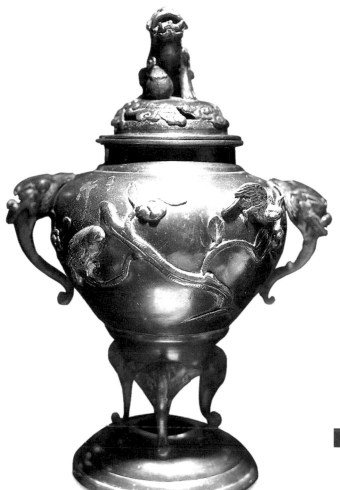

Perfume burner, China, c. 1850.

23

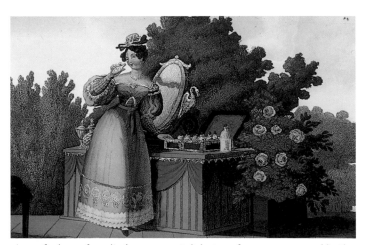

A profusion of vanity boxes containing perfumes appeared in the 19th century. This label, taken from one of them, shows a young woman at her dressing table. France, 19th century.

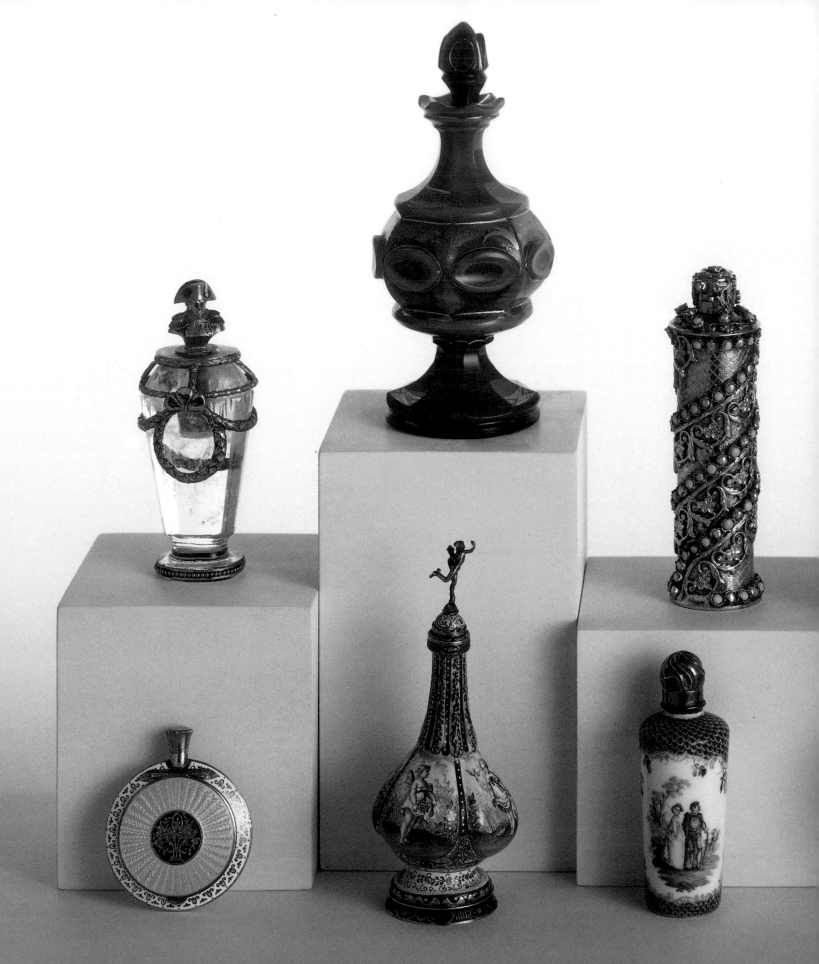

24

Top, left to right:
Carved quartz bottle with gilded mount and a bust of Napoleon I
as a stopper, France, c. 1810.
Dressing table bottle in marbled agate-like opaline, Georgenthal,
Bohemia, c. 1835.
Cylindrical silver gilt bottle with pearl and turquoise decoration,
Russia, c.1850.

Bottom, left to right:
Green enamel bottle, set in silver and bearing the stamp of the
master craftsman K.F., Vienna, Austria, 19th-20th century.
Enamel bottle, France, second half of the 19th century.
Porcelain and silver bottle, second half of the 19th century.

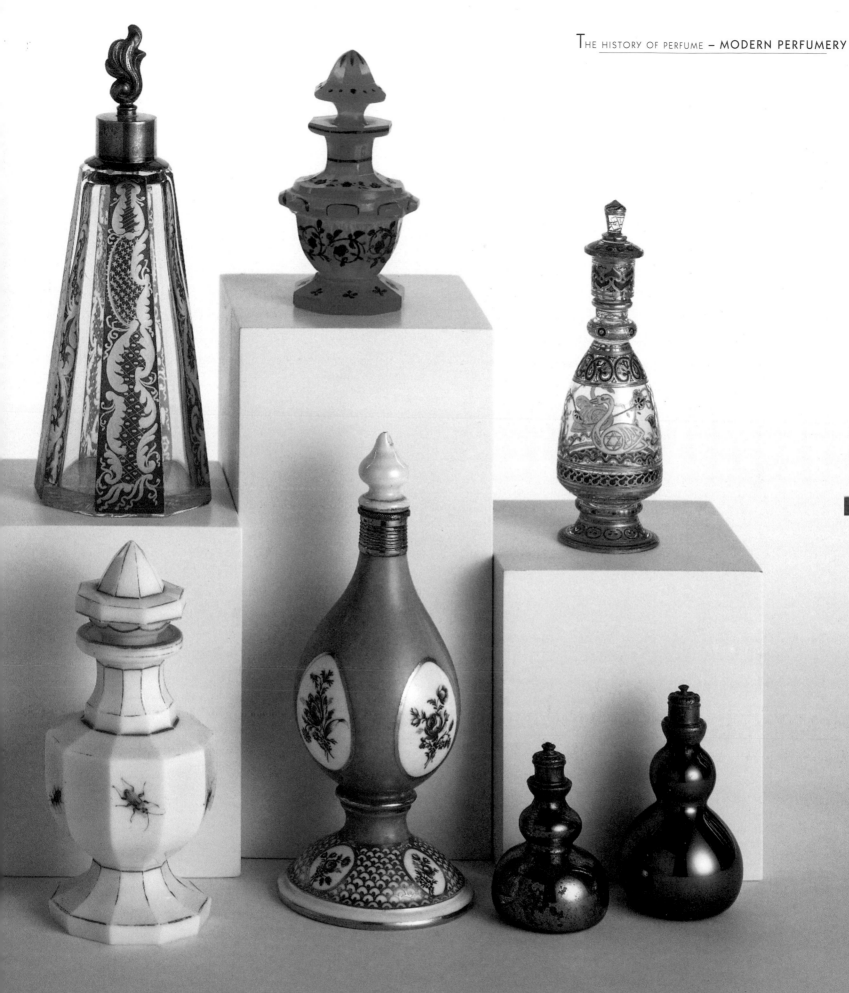

Top, left to right:
Glass and silver bottle, Bohemia, c. 1860.
Painted glass bottle, Bohemia, c. 1860.
Glass bottle made by the Lobmeyr factory,
Vienna, Austria, c. 1880.

Bottom, left to right:
Dressing table bottle in pure white opal glass, Neuwelt, Bohemia,
1835-1845.
Porcelain bottle, Vienna, Austria, 1770-1780.
Glass and pewter bottles, Germany, mid-18th century.

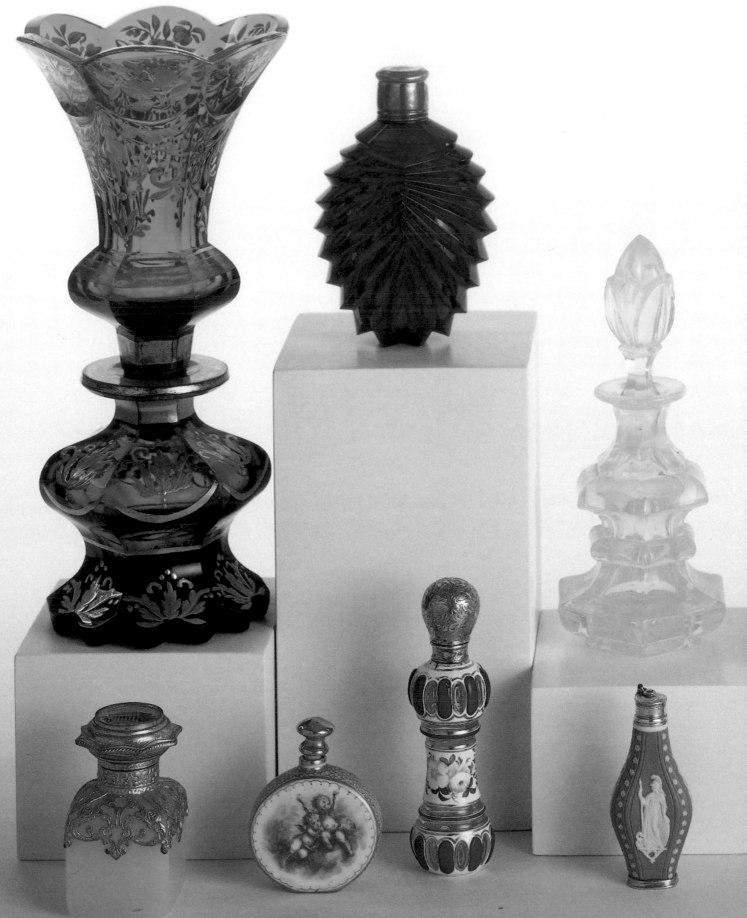

Top, left to right:
Faceted glass bottle with fine gold detailing and a stopper in the shape of a vase, Bohemia, c. 1840.
Crystal bottle, Bohemia, 19th century.
Stunningly colored bottle in faceted uranium glass, Bohemia, c. 1875.

Bottom, left to right:
Opal glass bottle with gilt decoration, France, 1870.
Porcelain bottle decorated with gold and painted with angels, Dresden, Germany, 19th century.
Bottle, Bohemia, c. 1850.
Jasper ware bottle, by Wedgwood or Turner, England, late 18th century.

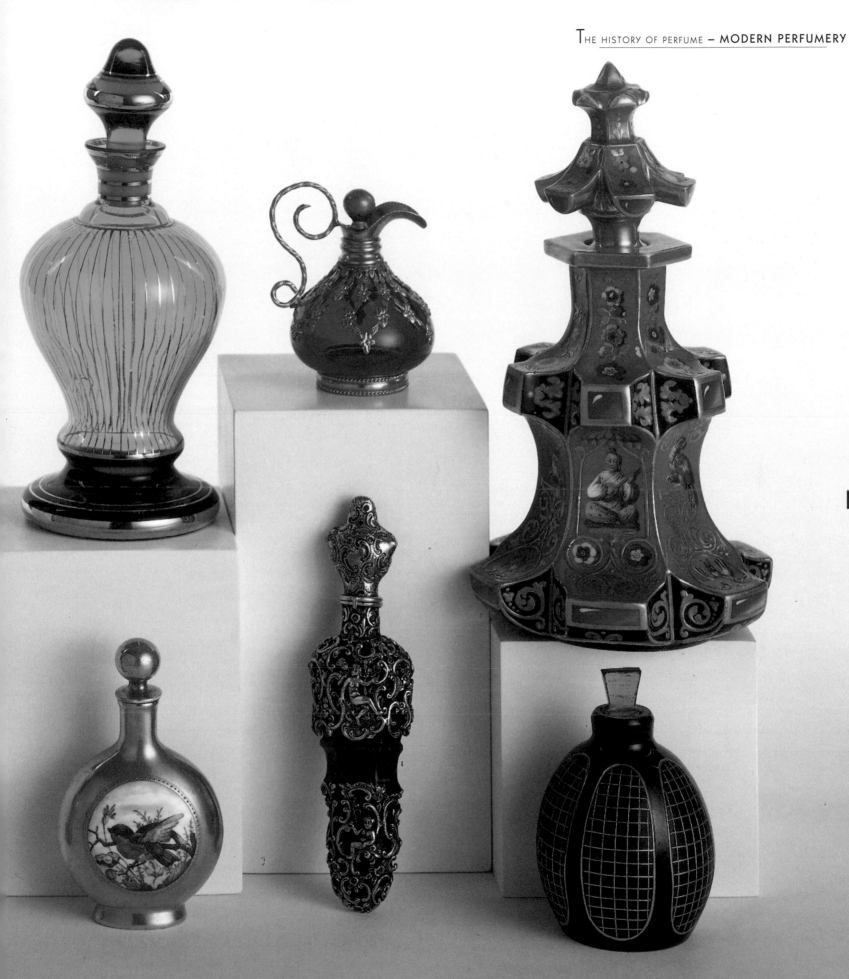

Top, left to right:
Glass bottle with gold design, Bohemia (?), 19th century (?).
Bronze burette, France, 1880.
Chinese-style porcelain dressing table bottle, Bohemia,
1834-1835.

Bottom, left to right:
Flattened round bottle in gold porcelain, painted with a robin on
a branch, England, 19th century.
Jasper bottle with finely carved silver mount studded with rubies
and sapphires, France, 18th-19th century.
Hyalite bottle, Bohemia, c. 1830.

Perfume in the Twentieth Century

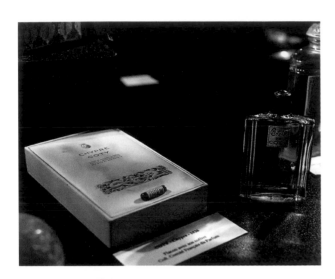

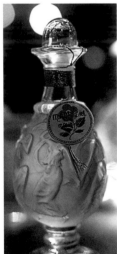

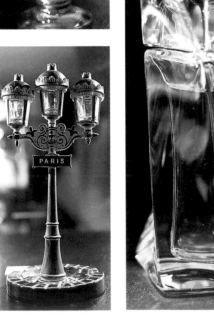

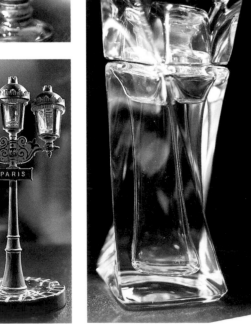

Above: **Chypre** *by Coty (1917).*
Left: **Madrigal** *by Molinard (1930).*
Below left: **Rue de la Paix** *by Corday (1952).*
Below right: **Magie** *by Lancôme (1950).*

By the end of the nineteenth century, the French perfume industry employed almost twenty thousand people, and a third of its turnover came from exports. Its success was honored at the 1900 World Fair in Paris, where the various exhibitors in the perfumery section were placed around a splendidly decorated central fountain. Art Nouveau masters were engaged to decorate the stands. So it was that Hector Guimard, designer of the entrances to the Paris Métro, came to create perfume bottles for Maillot and graphic designer Alfons Mucha became famous for his work with Houbigant.

There had been a gradual change in the perception of perfume. Quite apart from the fragrance itself, other elements such as the bottle, its packaging and its advertising gained importance. Perfume-makers soon joined forces with the greatest names in glass-making, graphic design and advertising. One of the most fruitful partnerships was that between the perfume-maker François Coty and René Lalique. It gave the glass-maker the opportunity to perfect his techniques and produce bottles for other perfume-makers like D'Orsay, Guerlain, Lubin, Molinard, Piver, Roger & Gallet and Volnay, as well as for Coty. Other glass-makers contributed to the blossoming of the bottle-making industry: first Baccarat, with their numerous creations for Guerlain (*Mitsouko, Shalimar* and *Coque d'Or* among others), Desprez, Houbigant and Caron (*Narcisse Noir*); and then the Brosse glassworks, which came to prominence in the Twenties with the superbly restrained lines of its bottle for *Chanel No.5* and the famous black sphere for Jeanne Lanvin's *Arpège*.

As for the perfumes themselves, they continued to evolve and improve, no longer in a period of ephemeral scents and rough approximations. François Coty's creations were the first to blend natural and artificially reproduced fragrances. *L'Origan*, launched in 1905, was the first great modern perfume. In 1917 he created *Chypre*, which engendered a family of fragrances bearing the same name and based on notes of oak moss, labdanum, patchouli or bergamot. The fragrances known as the Orientals blossomed, with the characteristic sweet, powdery, vanilla notes and dominant animal scents which are still evident today in *L'Heure Bleue* and *Shalimar* by Guerlain.

While synthetic products had revolutionized perfume blending by the end of the nineteenth century, perfumery itself was about to be turned upside down by the arrival of a new breed of perfume-maker, the couturier. Paul Poiret, already famous for having liberated women from their corsets, in 1911 was the first to have the idea of marketing a perfume to complement his lines of clothing. He christened his perfumes "*Les Parfums de Rosine,*" after his eldest daughter. However, although Poiret had understood the potential of house fragrances for a couturier, he did not push the idea to its logical commercial heights. This was left to the great Gabrielle Chanel, who in 1921 launched her own brand of perfume – for a first attempt, it was a master-stroke! The soon-to-be legendary *No.5*, created by Ernest Beaux, was the first perfume to employ aldehydes, powerful synthetic products which, as well as bringing their own fragrance to a blend, also made it very long-lasting. Lanvin would use them in turn for *Arpège.*

The Thirties saw the arrival of the leather group of fragrances, such as Lanvin's *Scandal* or Chanel's *Cuir de Russie,* with dry notes evoking the smell of leather and floral top notes. The floral group was augmented by perfumes like Worth's *Je Reviens* (1932), Caron's *Fleurs de Rocaille* (1933) and Jean Patou's *Joy* (1935). After the Second World War, the Chypre group was further developed with Rochas' *Femme* (1944), *Ma Griffe* by Carven and *Miss Dior* (1947). Nina Ricci's *L'Air du Temps* (1947) brought a new dimension to the floral family, as had Balmain's *Vent Vert* (1945). During the Fifties, French perfumery was at its peak. After Poiret, Chanel, Worth, Lanvin and Patou, all the major names in fashion turned to perfume – Elsa Schiaparelli (whose bottles, like their creator, possessed great charm), Pierre Balmain, Carven, Jacques Fath, Christian Dior, Nina Ricci, Hubert de Givenchy and so on. France also had the greatest perfume blenders – among them Edmond Roudnitska, who instigated another minor revolution with the use of hedione in his very attractive fragrance for men, *Eau Sauvage.* As well as seeing the launch of men's fragrances, it was also a time of increasing international competition with the arrival of perfumes from across the Atlantic.

Today, perfumery is more than ever a luxury industry which, like all other sectors of the economy, remains subject to certain constraints. The implacable logic of the marketing department is now as vital as the work of the "noses," who must try to attract increasingly demanding consumers. Twentieth-century perfumery has been driven by advances in the chemistry of fragrance; in the twenty-first century it will have to avoid fleeting trends and easy options and learn to assimilate technologies as revolutionary as genetics. All this, of course, without losing sight of the fact that perfumery remains an art.

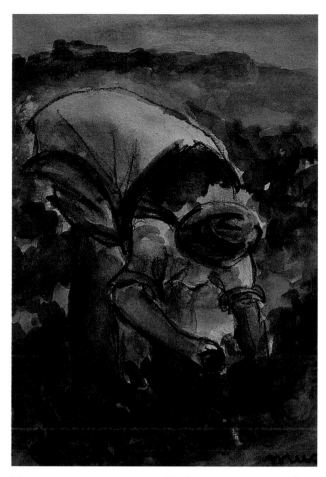

The art of modern perfumery lies in creating a harmonious blend of natural raw materials and synthetic products. The cultivation of lavender is therefore still a thriving industry.

The sense of smell was one which could not fail to fascinate an artist like Salvador Dali. The marriage between the two arts of perfumery and sculpture is beautifully realized in this bottle.

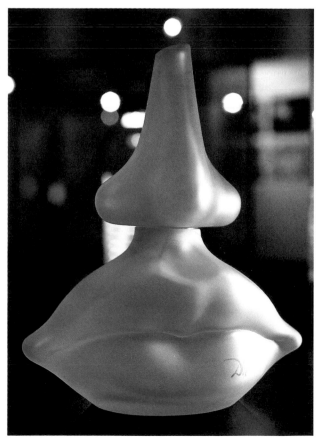

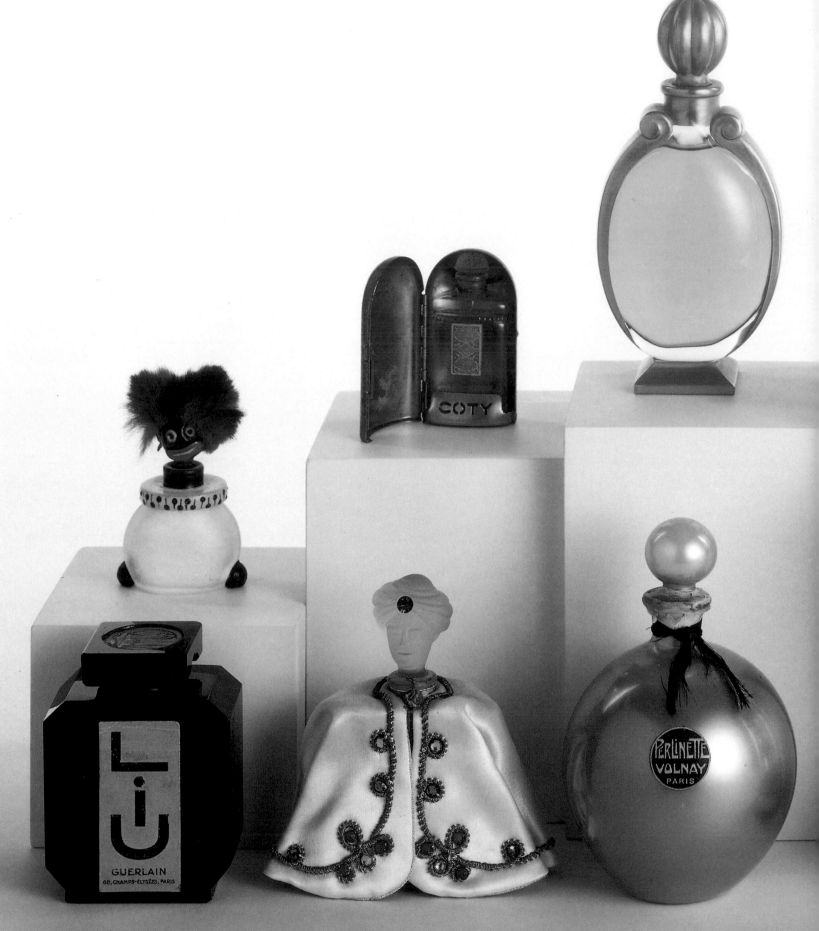

Top, left to right:
Golliwog by *De Vigny*. Bottle made by the Brosse glassworks using artificial fur, Paris, c. 1925. Based on the American doll featured in an English children's book, the bottle appeared at the same time as the first black jazz orchestra arrived in France.
L'Origan by Coty, Paris, 1905.
Rêve d'Or by *L.T. Piver*. Baccarat bottle and graphics both designed by Louis Süe, Paris, 1926.

Bottom, left to right:
Liu by *Guerlain*. Black and gold Baccarat bottle, Paris, c. 1929.
Prince Douka by *Marquay*. Glass bottle draped in a satin cape, with a head-shaped stopper wearing an Indian maharaja's turban set with an imitation diamond, Paris, 1951.
Perlinette by *Volnay*. Glass bottle with mother-of-pearl luster by the master glass-maker André Jolivet, manufactured by the Nesle Normandeuse glassworks, c. 1929.

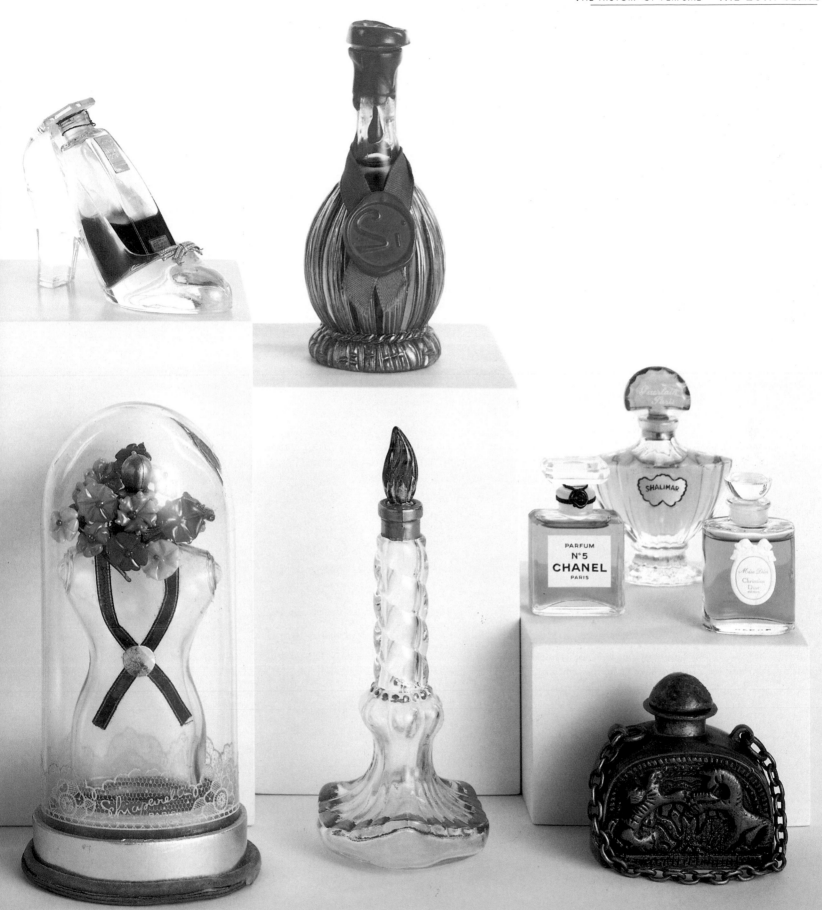

Top, left to right:
L'Aimant *by Coty. Bottle contained in a perspex shoe, Paris, c. 1940.*
Si *by Elsa Schiaparelli. Design inspired by a Chianti bottle, Paris, 1935.*
Chanel No.5, *Paris, 1921.*
Shalimar *by Guerlain, Paris, 1925.*
Miss Dior *by Christian Dior, Paris, 1947.*

Bottom, left to right:
Shocking *by Elsa Schiaparelli, Paris, 1936.*
Sleeping *by Elsa Schiaparelli. Baccarat bottle, Paris, 1938.*
Aladin Rosine *by Paul Poiret, Paris, 1923.*

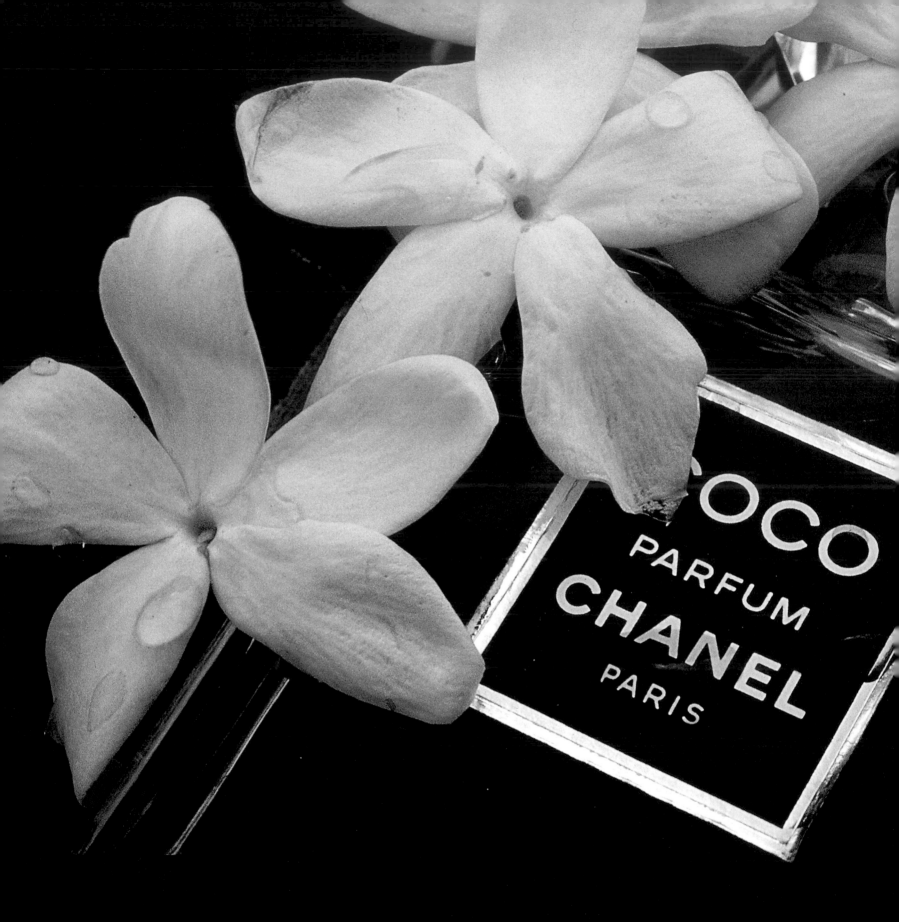

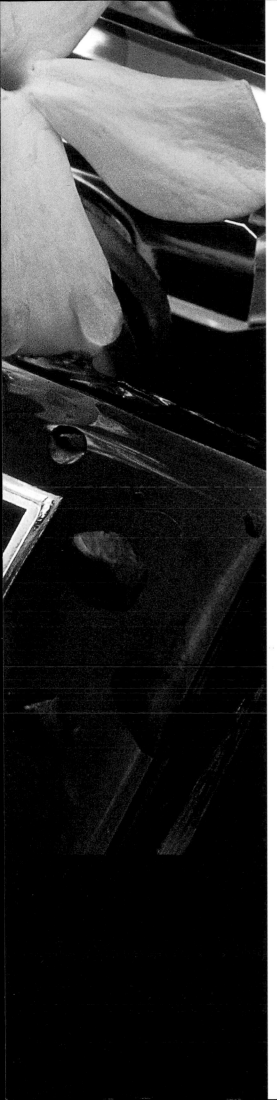

FROM PLANT TO PERFUME

It is interesting to note that those best qualified to talk about perfume – be they celebrated "noses," rose-growers from the plateaux around Grasse, devoted admirers of a single fragrance or producers of raw materials – invariably draw parallels between perfume, cookery and music. Their vocabulary is littered with terms such as notes, ingredients, resting times, scales, glazing and harmony. Of course, these apparently very different pursuits all combine training with intuition, respect for rules (scores, recipes or chemical formulae) with improvisations, and increasingly sophisticated techniques with traditional know-how.

The quality of raw materials is the starting point on the long journey from plant to perfume. A poor rose harvest, spoiled either by rain or heat, is as catastrophic for the perfume-maker as is a poor grape harvest for the wine-grower. Since poor products make for poor blends, the chemical processing involved is subject to the equally rigorous demands for quality, as are the methods of manufacture. It has taken man centuries to master the techniques of extracting essences from plants – advances in science have enabled him to recreate artificially what exists in nature or, better still, imbue a perfume with the smell of the sea, early morning dew or hot chocolate.

There is a common link between the woman harvesting the precious ylang-ylang flower at dawn in the Comoro Islands, the man watching the molecular structure of a wisteria flower appear on his computer screen and the factory worker tirelessly dusting each individual bottle of expensive perfume before packing them into boxes. It is this global chain which makes perfume such a prized commodity, at the same time exclusive and universal – something which remains particularly personal and yet responds to popular taste. Perfume is all of these things, but above all it is a question of the memories associated with it: the delicate, fresh smell of morning; the mysterious, heady aroma of a particular evening, which a lover will forever attempt to recapture; the trendy scent that wafts around every street corner; or the chance encounter with a nostalgic smell that takes us immediately back to the old-fashioned but delightful fragrances of our childhood.

Coco by Chanel, with its famous, Indian-grown jasmine.

The sperm whale excretes an odorous substance called ambergris, formed as a concretion in its intestines, which is not to be confused with amber, the odorless fossilized resin used in jewelry. Collected by fishermen at sea or beachcombers on the shore, ambergris is not a controllable resource, thereby making it a scarce raw material used only in expensive perfumes.

An internal gland of the beaver secretes castoreum, an oily substance with which the animal coats its fur for protection. Its characteristic odor of printer's ink is used in chypre perfumes with leather-tobacco notes.

RAW MATERIALS DERIVED FROM ANIMALS

People are often surprised to learn that a loveable little creature like the beaver plays an important part in the manufacture of their favorite perfume, or that the contents of a pouch removed from the belly of the musk deer can be used to make a fragrance more intense. It is reassuring to know that such practices, which were recently very widespread, are now strictly regulated to ensure the survival of the species concerned. However, these substances provide a useful understanding of the origins of synthetic products and the role that they play in the creation of a perfume.

AMBERGRIS

Ambergris, a concretion formed in the intestines of the sperm whale, is used by perfume-makers as a fixative for volatile fragrances. It is thought that large cephalopods, like cuttlefish and squid, are involved in its formation inside the whale's digestive tract – their beaks damage the lining of the intestine, which subsequently produces this paste-like secretion. Once freed, the ambergris is either immediately excreted or released during decomposition after the whale's natural death. Its use, therefore, does not endanger this highly protected species. Ambergris is lighter than water and floats freely on the ocean currents, refining itself naturally and fading with the combined action of the sun and water. It is collected on the high seas or after it has been washed ashore, and when it finally reaches the perfume-maker's laboratory it is light, porous and either pale grey or white in color. It is left to dry out for several months, after which time its nauseating fishy smell is replaced by the characteristic ambergris scent, with its hints of the seashore sometimes mixed with the merest suggestion of tea. It then undergoes a further several months of cold maceration in pure alcohol, resulting in a product of remarkable subtlety used as a fixative for high-quality perfumes. Ambergris comes in blocks or kidney-like shapes and can weigh from as little as a few ounces to over six hundred pounds. Its prohibitive price makes it a precious commodity and so it is used sparingly.

CASTOREUM

Castoreum is an odorous substance secreted by a pair of internal glands in the beaver – it is an oily, lustrous liquid that the animal uses to grease its fur in order to protect it from the elements. Once widespread throughout Europe, the beaver is now only found in North America and Russia and is hunted in January, when its fur is at its most beautiful. The pelts are the real prize of the hunt, with the glands regarded mainly as by-products. They weigh about four ounces and their size varies depending on the age of the animal. Castoreum is an excellent perfume fixative and is used in an alcoholic tincture, as a resinoid or as an absolute, imparting a warm, animal note similar to leather. Perfume-makers use Castoreum in Oriental, Chypre and men's fragrances.

MUSK

In perfumery terms, musk is the odorous secretion produced by a gland in the abdomen of the male musk deer. The gland is an oval or round pouch, between one and four inches in diameter, situated underneath the skin of the animal's belly, between the navel and the genitals. The musk deer is a ruminant belonging to the genus Moschus and lives on the high plateaux of central Asia and the Himalayas. It resembles a smaller, more primitive roe deer, weighs around twenty pounds and is a solitary, aggressive creature that marks its territory with pungent secretions. To protect the species, hunting has been forbidden and the export of musk is strictly regulated. Originally, the animal had to be killed in order to remove the glands. An attempt was then made at farming them, but it became evident that they stopped producing musk when in captivity. The least harmful method was thus deemed to be trapping and tranquillizing the deer during the rutting season, the period during which musk is secreted, and surgically removing the pouches before releasing the animal. It takes about twenty pouches to make one pound of musk which, once extracted from the pouch, forms a grainy powder like ground coffee but with an unbearably pungent smell of ammonia. After refining in an alcoholic tincture, the musk is transformed into a substance that lends a sensual, animal note and greater tenacity to a perfume. Musk was particularly fashionable in Ancient Greece and Rome, and again during the Renaissance when it was the favored substance of perfume-makers, along with ambergris and frankincense. Today, however, it is hardly ever used, as perfume-makers have replaced it with much less expensive synthetic musks.

CIVET

The civet is a small, solitary and very aggressive animal, weighing around 45 pounds and belonging to the Viverridae family. It is roughly the same size as a fox, with piercing eyes, long whiskers and tail, and grey-brown fur with black markings. The particular species of civet used in perfumery lives in the south-west of Ethiopia, where it is increasingly farmed. It has a crescent-shaped pouch close to the genitals which secretes viverreum, a soft and highly pungent substance, either beige or brown in color. This is surgically removed and once blended with other products, loses its pungency to impart a long-lasting sensuality and animal warmth to a perfume.

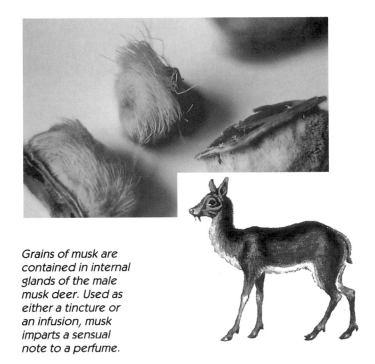

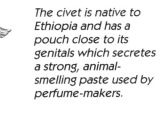

Grains of musk are contained in internal glands of the male musk deer. Used as either a tincture or an infusion, musk imparts a sensual note to a perfume.

35

The civet is native to Ethiopia and has a pouch close to its genitals which secretes a strong, animal-smelling paste used by perfume-makers.

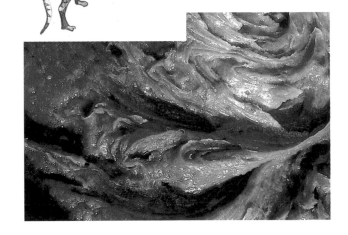

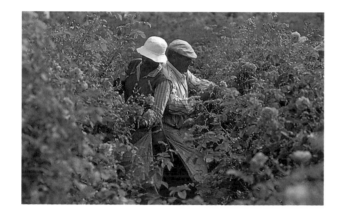

Jasmine. In Grasse, where all flowers are called by their proper names, it is simply known as "the flower."

In Grasse, the May rose is harvested only once a year over a short three-week period. Just as with the grape harvest, some years have a better yield than others.

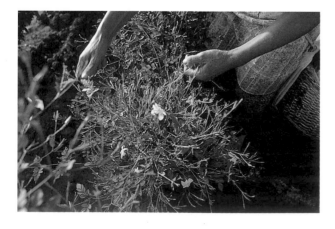

Jasmine picking begins at dawn. The flower is so light that only about one and a half pounds can be gathered per hour. About four thousand flowers are needed to make one pound of jasmine.

RAW MATERIALS DERIVED FROM PLANTS

While flowers are the plant products most widely employed in perfumery, they are not the only ones – other raw materials derived from plants, regularly put to different uses in our daily lives, are also important tools of the perfume-maker's trade.

FLOWERS, PETALS, BUDS AND SHOOTS

Though the link between flowers and perfume today seems an obvious one, perfumery's use of floral raw materials was not a development that took place overnight. Great imagination and ingenuity were required to capture in a bottle the quintessential complexity and magic contained within a plant.

ROSE

Of all flowers, the rose has undoubtedly been the favorite among perfume lovers for over three thousand years. Homer wrote of the rose oil, made by macerating the petals in olive oil, which Aphrodite smoothed over Hector's body. Islamic perfume-makers were the first to distil the petals of the damask rose and the Persian town of Shiraz was renowned from the eighth century onwards for the rose-water which it continued to export to Europe, India and China until the seventeenth century. Besides its culinary and medicinal uses, rose water was highly prized by western perfume-makers from the Renaissance right up to the nineteenth century. The sultans of Persia took sophistication a stage further by having their mattresses stuffed with the precious petals.

The perfume industry uses two botanical varieties of rose from among the hundreds of known species: *Rosa centifolia*, also called the May or Provence rose, found in Grasse and Morocco; and *Rosa damascena*, the damask rose, grown in Bulgaria and Turkey. The Grasse *centifolia* is treated by extraction with volatile solvents to produce a concrete and then an absolute, whereas the Moroccan *centifolia* and Turkish *damascena* undergo either solvent extraction or steam distillation, the latter technique resulting in an essential oil (see page 51). In the case of the Bulgarian *damascena*, only steam distillation is used.

The rose harvest is a particularly delicate process and its worst enemy is the sun, for although the rose's perfume is stronger in the heat of midday, it is also less sweet. The concentration of volatile scents is at its highest at about 8:30 am and picking therefore begins at dawn, moving from flower to flower as quickly as possible. An experienced picker can gather between ten and eighteen pounds of petals per hour, with the most productive workers harvesting over one hundred pounds per day. While this may initially seem a huge figure, bear in mind that it takes about two and a half tons of flowers to produce one single pound of essence. This means that it would take over twenty-four hours of picking to produce a single ounce of essential oil. This oil consists of almost three hundred component molecules, some of them difficult to identify, which explains why science has not yet succeeded in accurately reproducing the subtlety of this natural base. Yet this is no cause for complaint – quite apart from the magnificent sight of the rose fields themselves, extraordinarily beautiful fragrances such as *Joy* by Jean Patou and Yves Saint Laurent's *Paris* owe their beauty to the rose.

JASMINE

The list of fragrant notes associated with jasmine is endless – flowery, warm, animal, spicy, fruity, rich and so on. It is such a central pillar of the perfume-making business that in Grasse, where all flowers are called by their proper names, jasmine is known simply as "the flower."

The species used in perfumery is *Jasminum grandiflorum*, a shrub probably native to Persia and central Asia which flowers from August to October. It was introduced into Grasse in around 1560 by Spanish sailors and came into widespread commercial use in the nineteenth and early twentieth centuries. Despite the fact that major names like Patou and Chanel have recently signed agreements with jasmine growers, there are today only a few jasmine farms left in operation in Grasse, each covering less than twenty-five acres. Jasmine is also grown in Egypt, Italy, Morocco and particularly India, where labor costs are significantly lower. Whereas today's production levels are relatively low, at the turn of the century two hundred tons of jasmine were produced annually, and between 1930 and 1940 this figure rose to almost two thousand tons. Bearing in mind that four thousand flowers are needed to make just one pound of jasmine, it is difficult to imagine the number of workers and fields such a vast production must have involved. As with the rose, harvesting takes place before dawn so that dew and heat do not spoil the precious white flowers, which are picked individually. A good worker gathers about one and a half pounds of jasmine per hour and the flowers are taken to the factory as quickly as possible to be treated by extraction – seven hundred and fifty pounds of flowers are required to produce one pound of absolute.

In the Thirties, some perfumes contained up to ten per cent absolute essence of jasmine, but today concentrations are lower, reaching at most only one or two per cent. Jasmine is the most widely used white flower in perfume manufacture and, according to blenders, no great perfume is made without it. It is at the heart of many classic perfumes, such as Chanel's ever popular *No.5*, *Joy* by Patou, *Arpège* by Lanvin, *Fleur de Fleurs* by Nina Ricci and Van Cleef's *First*.

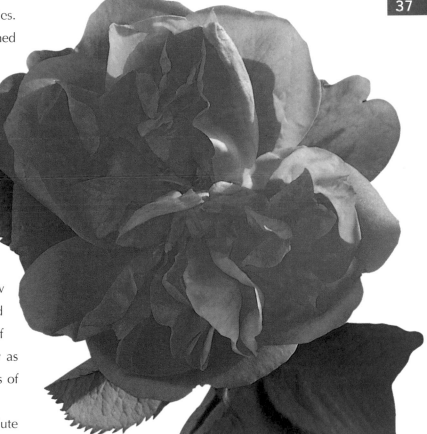

Rosa centifolia, the May rose, is one of two species of rose used by perfume-makers. Each year, it yields a few pounds of the most expensive absolute essence in the world.

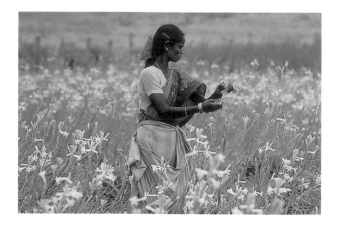

The tuberose blooms all year round in Karnataka state in south-eastern India, but the flowers harvested in July and August provide the best fragrant tones.

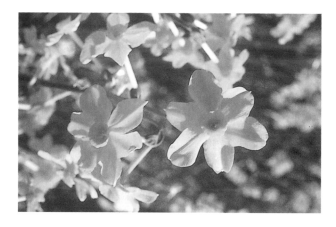

The narcissus used in perfume manufacture grows on mountains above three thousand feet. Treatment of the flowers and stems produces an absolute essence which blends very well with both green and animal notes.

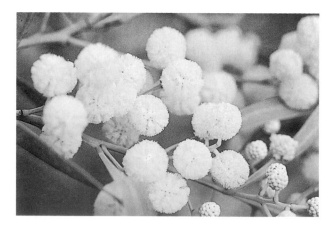

Mimosa, a winter flower with no petals, has only very rarely been used as the main note in a perfume. Its absolute essence, with powdery, warm and flowery tones, is added to floral compositions.

TUBEROSE

The tuberose, *Polianthes tuberosa*, is a headily-scented flower native to Mexico which was introduced into France in the seventeenth century and cultivated principally in Grasse. It was particularly popular at the court of Louis XIV, the Sun King, where the great beauties of the time wore them on their bodices. Today, it is grown mainly in Karnataka State in south-eastern India, where it flowers all year round. It has a rich, warm scent with hints of balsam which perfume-makers use in Oriental blends, such as Christian Dior's *Poison*.

NARCISSUS

The narcissus, an alpine flower with an unmistakable perfume, grows in the meadows of the Jura, the Alps and the Massif Central. The species used in perfume manufacture is the relatively rare, May-flowering *Narcissus poeticus* or pheasant's-eye. The flowers are treated by solvent extraction along with the stems and leaves, producing an absolute that echoes the scent of the flower with an additional hint of foliage. It is a very expensive raw material: the flowers cost about one dollar per pound and about twelve hundred pounds are needed to make just one pound of the absolute. Narcissus imparts a very intense note to a perfume.

MIMOSA

The mimosa is a native of Australia but has adapted well to the Mediterranean climate, lending a delightfully bright and summery color to the hills of the Riviera from late January to early March. Its golden spheres are not made up of petals but rather of stamens. This explains why the flowers are so fragile, making it impossible to keep mimosa for more than twenty-four hours after picking. Both the flowers and leaves are treated, resulting in an absolute that replicates the scent of the flower, at the same time sweet and "ticklish." While mimosa is a flower that enjoys great popularity in Britain, it has never really been used to provide the dominant note in a perfume.

ORANGE FLOWER

The orange flower is a symbol of virginity. In Grasse, couples who marry during the flowering season in April and May are traditionally given garlands made from them. The flower comes from the bitter orange, *Citrus aurantium amara*, a tree native to southern China but introduced into Mediterranean countries in Roman times. Distillation results in an essence called neroli and the water produced during this process is the renowned orange flower water. Although an absolute essence of orange flower can be obtained by solvent extraction, the yield is very low, with about a thousand pounds of flowers producing about a pound of neroli. The leaves and young branches of the bitter orange are also treated, creating an essence known as petitgrain, while the zest of the orange itself produces an essence called bigarade when processed by the expression method.

LAVENDER

Invariably associated with Provence, but also less romantically with the hygienic smell of detergents and soap powders, lavender is rarely considered a fashionable ingredient by the modern perfume industry. Considering that it possesses such an interesting tonality of fragrance, this is rather unfair treatment. Contrary to popular belief, the beauty of the hillsides in the Lubéron and the plateaux around Manosque comes not from lavender but from a hybrid species called lavandin, or French lavender. The true lavender used in perfume manufacture is a lower-growing plant with finer stems, the cost of which is much higher and which grows above three thousand feet in the Alps, but more commonly in Britain. At the turn of the century, the British were famous for their single-fragrance creations based on lavender: Atkinson's *English Lavender* (1910), the first eau de toilette for men, and Yardley's *Old English Lavender* (1913), that essential accessory to the tweed suit. These were both to be succeeded by Caron's *Pour un Homme* (1934). Although today's perfume-makers would probably not attempt the launch of a lavender-scented fragrance because of its inevitable associations with clean laundry, they nevertheless use it as a top note in men's eaux de toilette to add freshness to the blend.

YLANG-YLANG

Cananga odorata forma genuina, better known as the ylang-ylang, produces a flower that evokes the sweet, sticky heat of the tropics. It is a native of the Philippines but became established in the Comoro Islands and Madagascar, where it is still grown today. In the wild, the ylang-ylang is a tree with twisting branches which can reach between eighty and ninety-five feet in height. When cultivated, however, it is pruned to about six feet, accentuating its contorted form. Worn in the hair by the women of Manila and once used to perfume harems, the flower is symbolic of sensual pleasure and seduction. The note is a favorite with blenders, having great immediate "lift", which later turns more floral and powdery, and possessing great tenacity.

Also noteworthy here are the jonquil (*Narcissus odorus*), one of the first flowers of the year which has a delicate, penetrating scent, as well as the hyacinth (*Hyacinthus orientalis*), another plant which grows in woodland glades, whose bell-shaped flowers produce a highly refreshing absolute

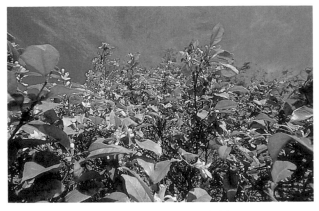

The flowers of the bitter orange tree yield an essence called neroli, named after the sixteenth-century Duchess Orsini de Neroli, who was infatuated with the fragrance. While it is a pure, fresh substance, used as a base in all eaux de Cologne, neroli nevertheless has warm, animal tones.

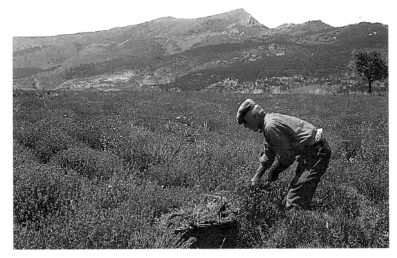

Although lavender was highly valued at the turn of the century, it is scarcely ever used today because of its extensive use in the manufacture of washing powders and air fresheners.

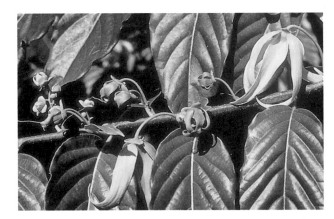

The ylang-ylang, or "flower of flowers" as perfume-makers call it, comes from a tree native to the Philippines. It is picked when the yellow of the flowers is at its most intense and a slight red coloration appears in the middle of the petals.

essence. The use of these two flowers in perfume manufacture has practically disappeared as they have been replaced by blends that replicate their fragrance. Then there are the helichrysum flowers, which once dried yield a warm, spicy essence with hints of tobacco and leather. The cassie, a tall-growing thorny bush of the wattle family with yellow flowers similar to mimosa, produces a warm and delicate absolute which blends well with orris and violet. The fragrant olive *(Osmanthus fragrans)*, an ornamental tree known to the Chinese for two and a half thousand years, is today used to create a beautifully scented absolute with fruity-floral tones. Finally, there is broom and the French marigold *(Tagetes glandulifera or T. patula)*, sometimes known as "the carnation of India," which yields a subtle essence, both flowery and fruity and reminiscent of foliage.

There are, however, some interesting omissions from this list. In the early years of this century, some two hundred tons of carnations were processed annually in Grasse whereas today hardly any are grown, as synthetic products are used to reproduce the fragrance artificially. The lilac has fared little better, but this is because extraction has proved almost entirely unsuccessful. Anyone who recognizes the heady scent of honeysuckle or lily of the valley will doubtless be surprised to learn that these two plants are completely immune to any of the distillation or extraction processes. It is almost as though nature, angered by so much theft, has given herself some small measure of revenge.

ROOTS AND RHIZOMES

Although the flowers of some plants do not respond at all to extraction, their roots and rhizomes often provide valuable essences that are widely used in perfume manufacture.

ORRIS

Of the three hundred known species of iris, only two are used in perfumery: *Iris pallida* and *Iris florentina*. They are grown mainly in Morocco and in the region around Florence, but it is in fact the roots and not the flower which are valued by perfume-makers. Their scent differs from that of the flower and, once treated, bears a resemblance to the smell of violets. The rhizome (or orris root) is harvested three years after planting and dried for a further three years to ensure an optimum yield of perfume. The roots are then ground, diluted in water and distilled. It is a long and costly process: one ton of orris root produces four pounds of extremely expensive essential oil with a beautifully subtle and powerful scent. It imparts a heavy, woody and long-lasting floral note reminiscent of the kind of old-fashioned face powders our grandmothers might have worn. When a perfume carries the scent of irises it is, therefore, one whose principal ingredient is orris root.

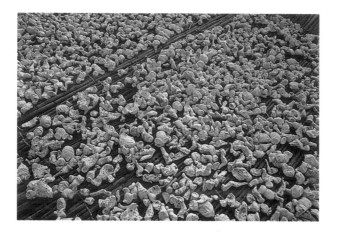

For perfume-makers, the important part of the iris is the root. The best are grown, and later dried, in Florence.

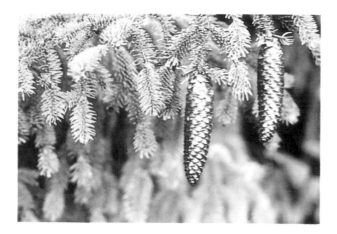

Several varieties of pine tree yield an essence or a resinoid of pine, which is used mainly in industrial perfumery.

40

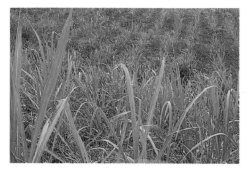

The rhizomes of other plants used in perfume making include ginger *(Zingiber officinalis)*, which is grown in China, India, Liberia and Jamaica. Ginger is best known for its culinary uses, although a distilled essence is also employed in perfumery. Lovage *(Levisticum officinalis)* is a tall-growing herb, cultivated since Roman times, whose roots are distilled to provide a warm and powerful essence that is especially effective in woody, spicy or Oriental blends. Until the practice was prohibited by law, perfume-makers also used the roots of the valerian *(Valeriana officinalis)* and the costus or spiral flag, from Kashmir, both of which produced a very pronounced animal note after distillation. Lastly, there is vetiver. Known botanically as *Andropogon squarrosus* and to the Indians as *cuscus*, it is a grass-like plant grown primarily in Haiti, India, Indonesia and Réunion. Distillation of the roots yields an essential oil often used as a basis for extracting acetate of vetiver, rather than in its pure state.

The vetiver grown on Réunion first appeared on the island in 1850. Under the name of Bourbon vetiver, it has since become one of the island's most valuable crops.

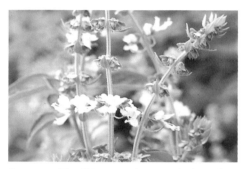

Provençal basil is one of two varieties of the herb used in perfume manufacture.

LEAVES, HERBS AND STEMS

GERANIUM

There are two hundred and fifty species of geranium but only three, grown on the high plateaux of Réunion and in the Nile delta in Egypt, are used in perfume manufacture. Essential oil of geranium, obtained by distillation of the leaves, produces a pleasant floral note sometimes likened to rose. Not surprisingly, the essence contains molecules also found in rose oil.

PATCHOULI

The emblematic perfume of hippy "flower power" in the Seventies, patchouli is made from the dried leaves of *Pogostemon cablin*, widely grown in Indonesia. It has a highly individual scent, with camphor-like, earthy and woody overtones.

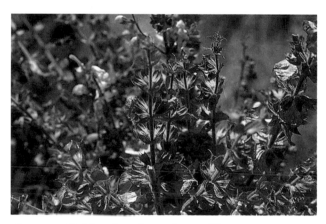

Clary sage (Salvia sclarea) *produces either an essence or an absolute well-suited to men's fragrances.*

VIOLET

Only the leaves of *Viola odorata* are used for perfume, solvent extraction resulting in a particularly verdant floral absolute. The violet was highly valued during the early days of modern perfumery (Roger & Gallet's *Vera Violetta* of 1892 and Houbigant's *Violette Pourpre* of 1907) and is now often used as a fixative for other ingredients.

It is the leaves, rather than the flowers, of the geranium which are employed in perfumery. The best varieties are unlike the familiar garden cultivars and are grown on Réunion as well as in Egypt.

MYRTLE

The young branches of *Myrtus communis* are treated to produce an essence which is used in small quantities to bring a herbal note to a perfume. This Mediterranean tree used to be associated with Venus and was an emblem of happy lovers. The Romans flavored their wines with myrtle branches and leaves and also added the leaves to their baths.

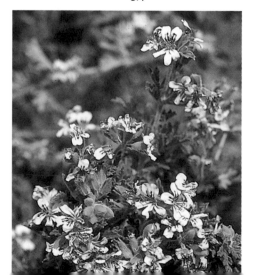

41

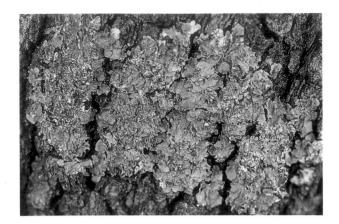

Oak moss yields an absolute essence which is vital to any chypre blend.

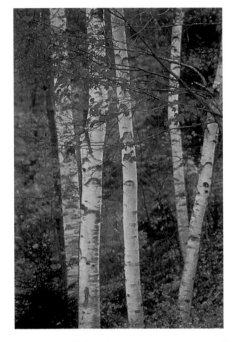

Essence of birch has a very pronounced smell of leather.

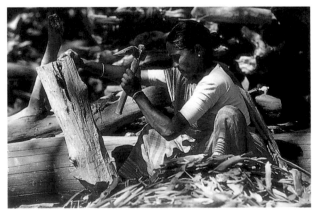

Sandalwood has been highly valued in India since ancient times and is used in religious fumigation ceremonies, cabinet-making and, after distillation, perfumery.

Among the other plants used in perfume-making, a few deserve mention here: wormwood, a wild plant which yields an aromatic, herbal essence; basil; bay; citronella, a tall-growing herb cultivated in India, Indonesia and China; cypress; eucalyptus; fennel; marjoram; maté, a small South American tree whose leaves are chewed by the native Indians; mint; origanum; parsley; pine; common and clary sage; tarragon; thyme; tobacco; and verbena.

WOOD, BARK, MOSSES AND LICHENS

These materials have been used since ancient times for fumigation ceremonies and play an important role in modern perfumery as ingredients in woody and chypre compositions.

CINNAMON
With an aroma made familiar by mulled wine and various cakes and pastries, cinnamon has been a highly prized spice since the sixteenth century and is used in perfumery in the form of an essential oil. The species employed is *Cinnamomum zeylanicum*, grown in Ceylon, Malaysia and the Seychelles, and whose strong, sweet essence is vital to any Oriental fragrance.

SANDALWOOD
Both the wood and the roots of *Santalum album* are treated by steam distillation to produce a warm and expansive essential oil – *Amazone* by Hermès, *Jicky* by Guerlain and *Métal* by Paco Rabanne are just three among the numerous perfumes made with essence of sandalwood. The most valued wood comes from the state of Karnataka in India although, because their forests are currently protected, no official sandalwood growing business exists there.

MOSSES
Solvent extraction of oak moss *(Evernia prunastri)*, harvested in temperate climates from winter to early spring, and common tree moss *(Evernia furfurcea)* produces absolutes which are indispensable in verdant chypre perfumes such as Dior's *Miss Dior*, *Quartz* by Molyneux and *Kouros* by Yves Saint Laurent.

Rosewood is another example of a raw material in this category. Its essence is obtained by distillation of the wood of *Aniba rosaedora*, a tree grown in Brazil, Peru and Guyana. It is a principal ingredient, along with essence of birch, in perfumes belonging to the leather group. Other woody blends are composed with the essences of thuya and cedar.

RESINS, GUMS AND BALSAMS

Resins, gums, gum resins and balsams, though little known outside the industry, are of great value to perfume-makers. These substances are exuded by certain plants either naturally or as a result of tapping. These four terms are not interchangeable as each substance has its own specific qualities. Each has a different degree of solubility, and resins, unlike gums, contain a fragrance.

SIAM BENZOIN

This resin is obtained by tapping the trunk of *Styrax tonkinensis*, a bush grown in Laos and Vietnam. Solvent extraction results in what is called a resinoid, used by perfume-makers to give depth to the base notes of a composition.

LABDANUM

The leaves of *Cistus ladaniferus*, a bush native to the Mediterranean basin, exude this gum resin, whose absolute is of particular value in chypre and Oriental blends.

FRANKINCENSE

Boswellia carterii or *B. saera* is a wild bush native to Somalia and southern Arabia. Its essence, obtained by distillation, is used as a top note and lends a hint of spice to a perfume. Its resinoid, obtained by extraction, has a heavier tone and is used as a middle or base note in Oriental or woody blends.

GALBANUM

This gum resin is obtained by tapping the trunk of the *Ferula galbaniflua*, a herbaceous plant grown principally in Iran. Once it has been treated by either steam distillation or solvent extraction, galbanum provides a green note, marvellously captured in *Fidji* by Guy Laroche and Balmain's *Vent Vert*.

MYRRH

The most valuable of the Magi's gifts, myrrh is a resin derived from the bush *Commiphora myrrha*. The note produced by either its essence or its resinoid evokes the scent of the forest floor. It is used by perfume-makers in blends of the chypre and fern groups.

Also worth mentioning are elemi, obtained from a gum resin exuded by the Manillan elemi, a large tree native to the Philippines, and opopanax, whose essence and resinoid are reminiscent of myrrh and are used in Guerlain's

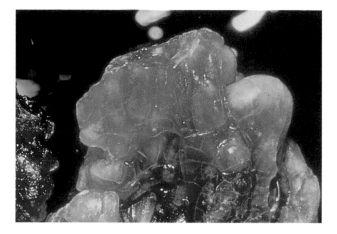

Siam benzoin resin.

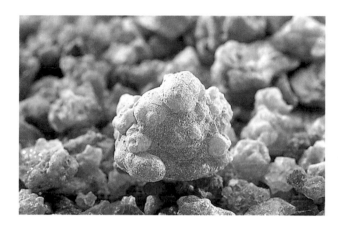

Opopanax resin.

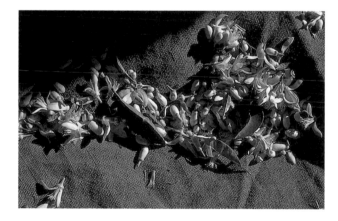

The leaves of the cistus exude a gum called labdanum.

Myrrh resin.

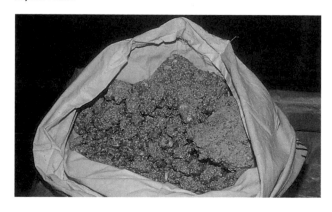

43

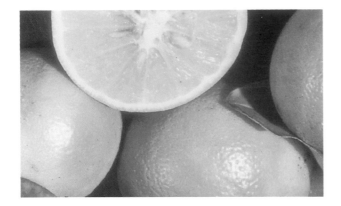

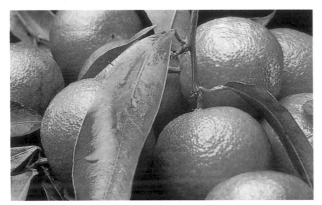

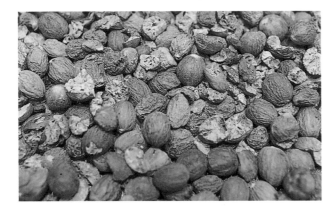

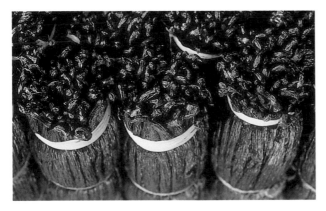

From top: *The fruits of* Citrus bergamia *(bergamot) and* Citrus reticulata *(mandarin), the nut contained in the fruit of* Myristica fragrans *(nutmeg), and the seed pod produced by* Vanilla planifolia *(vanilla).*

famous *Shalimar*. Tolu, a balsam derived from a tree grown in Bolivia and Venezuela, has a sweet tone best suited to Oriental blends. Interestingly, myrrh, frankincense, galbanum and opopanax are all ingredients that featured in early perfumes made by the ancient Egyptians.

FRUITS AND CITRUS ZESTS

With their high water content, the fragrance of most fruits is too dilute to be exploited in perfume manufacture. Only fruits whose zests contain aromatic oils and fruits which can be dried are used. These are known in the perfume trade as Cituses (lemons, mandarins, oranges, etc.) and are used in all blends of eau de Cologne.

LEMON

The fruit of *Citrus limon,* which is principally cultivated in Italy, Florida, South America and the Ivory Coast, produces an essential oil through expression (see page 53) of the zest. This oil is then used as a refreshing top note in perfumes.

ORANGE

The zest of both the bitter and sweet orange *(Citrus aurantium amara* and *C. aurantium dulcis* respectively) are employed to obtain an essential oil, used to great effect in tonic perfumes and eaux de Cologne.

MANDARIN

Native to China, where its fruits were once offered to the provincial governors, or mandarins, *Citrus reticulata* yields an essential oil after expression of the zest.

GRAPEFRUIT

Citrus paradisi provides essential oil of grapefruit, which is mainly produced in Israel and in the United States. It has only recently come to be used as an ingredient in perfume manufacture and often acts as a modifier in citrus blends.

There is also the bergamot, the inedible fruit of *Citrus bergamia,* which resembles a large orange and whose highly volatile essence gives lift to a perfume. Citron, derived from the fruit of *Citrus medica,* was widely used in the eighteenth and nineteenth centuries but has been ignored by today's perfume-makers. Essence of lime, however, from the plant *Citrus aurantifolia,* is still used in sports fragrances and men's eaux de toilette, as well as in Coca Cola!

ANISE AND STAR ANISE

Essence of anise is obtained by distillation of the small dried fruits of the European herb *Pimpinella anisum*. The essential oil of star anise is obtained through distillation of the characteristically shaped fruits of *Illicium verum*, a large tree native to Vietnam and southern China. The note is used in refreshing blends.

NUTMEG

The nutmeg is the intensely bitter-tasting fruit of the evergreen nutmeg tree, known to botanists as *Myristica fragrans,* grown largely in the East and West Indies. When picked, this hard little fruit, about the size of an apricot, has a red, fibrous skin known as mace. Both elements of the fruit are used in perfume manufacture, imparting a spicy scent to modern eaux de Cologne and fragrances for men.

VANILLA

Vanilla planifolia is a climbing plant of the orchid family, native to Mexico but introduced into Madagascar, Réunion and the Comoro Islands in the eighteenth century. It produces yellow or greenish-white flowers and slightly flattened seed pods lined with hairs which secrete a yellow, viscous substance with a warm, sweet, balsamic smell. Vanilla yields a powerfully scented essence with fixative qualities which has been used in numerous perfumes, most notably those by Guerlain.

Other fruits include cloves, the pistils of a tree which grows wild in Malaysia, Madagascar and Zanzibar, whose spicy essence is of great importance in perfume manufacture and, when blended with essence of rose, reproduces the scent of carnations. Anybody who recognizes the smell of gin will be familiar with the scent of juniper berries. The essence they produce has a fruity, woody and conifer-like fragrance. Lastly, distillation of the berries of the allspice plant, *Pimenta officinalis*, results in an essence with spicy, balsamic tones, used in small quantities by perfume-makers in Oriental and carnation-type floral blends.

SEEDS

This category of raw materials provides further evidence of the links between perfume-making and the art of cookery.

CARDAMOM

The seeds of the *Elettaria cardamomum*, a plant native to India, Ceylon, Indonesia and Central America, yield an aromatic and slightly fruity essential oil which brings great lift to perfume blends.

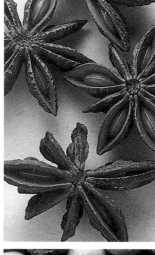
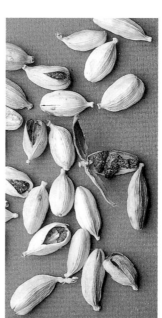
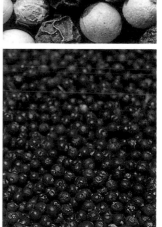
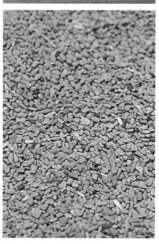
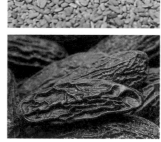

Clockwise from top right: *Star anise, peppercorns, juniper berries, tonka beans, fenugreek seeds and cardamom pods.*

CORIANDER

Essential oil of coriander is obtained by distillation of the seeds of *Coriandrum sativum*, a herb grown in the Ukraine, Hungary and North Africa, and imparts a peppery note with suggestions of chocolate.

CUMIN

The dried seeds of *Cuminum cyminum*, a herb native to the Mediterranean basin and India, are distilled to produce an essential oil which is employed in aromatic woody and fern blends. As its spicy aniseed tones are very strong, only small quantities are used.

FENUGREEK

Extraction of the seeds of this herb, native to India and Asia Minor, yields a powerful resinoid whose fragrance is reminiscent of walnut and celery. Although it played an important role in the perfumery of antiquity and the Islamic world, it has now fallen into disuse.

PEPPER

The bunched berries of the climbing shrub *Piper nigrum* are green when they first appear, harvested when they ripen to red, and then later turn brown. Essence of pepper is used primarily in fragrances for men.

TONKA BEAN

The seeds contained in the fruit of *Dipterix odorata*, which grows in Guyana and Brazil, are treated by extraction to produce an absolute used as a base note in spicy, tobacco and oriental blends.

46

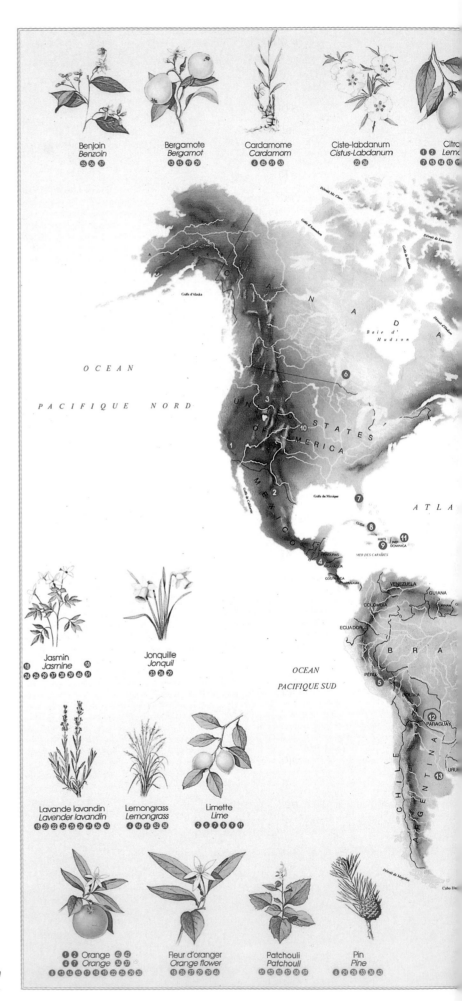

Map showing the origin of the main raw materials used in perfume manufacture, courtesy of Givaudan Roure.

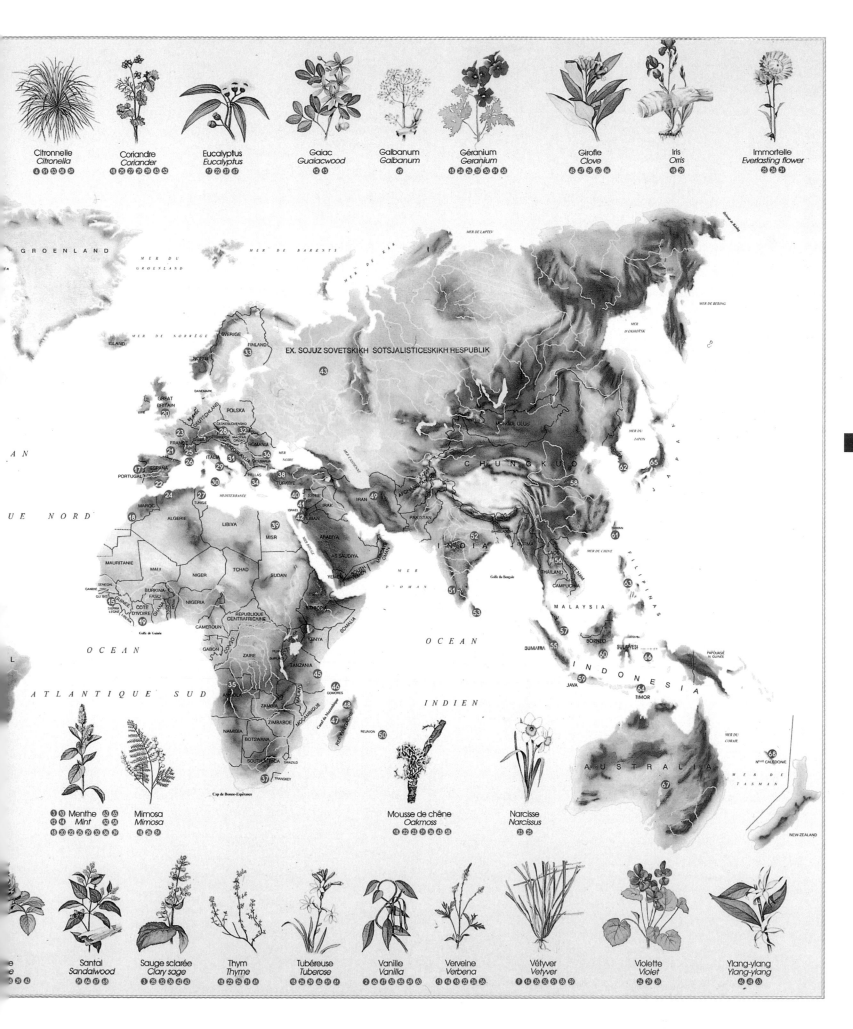

Citronnelle
Citronella

Coriandre
Coriander

Eucalyptus
Eucalyptus

Gaïac
Guaiacwood

Galbanum
Galbanum

Géranium
Geranium

Girofle
Clove

Iris
Orris

Immortelle
Everlasting flower

Menthe
Mint

Mimosa
Mimosa

Mousse de chêne
Oakmoss

Narcisse
Narcissus

Santal
Sandalwood

Sauge sclarée
Clary sage

Thym
Thyme

Tubéreuse
Tuberose

Vanille
Vanilla

Verveine
Verbena

Vétyver
Vetyver

Violette
Violet

Ylang-ylang
Ylang-ylang

SYNTHETIC MATERIALS

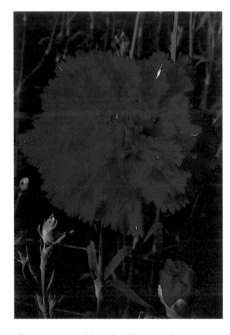

There are between two and three thousand fragrances manufactured synthetically, including the lilac, which would never have appeared in perfume without the advances made in chemistry.

Once treated by distillation, the carnation is now reproduced by synthesis.

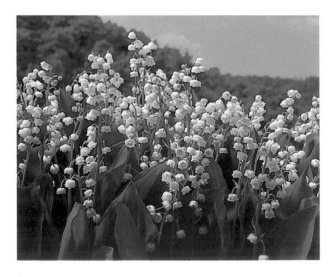

Lily of the valley is immune to any form of distillation or extraction, but is magically replicated in perfumes by the use of hydroxycitronellal, linalol and farnesol.

Chanel No.5 would not exist without aldehydes, and without the use of hedione, Edmond Roudnitska could never have created *Eau Sauvage*. These claims still come as a surprise to some, despite the fact that the use of synthetic products in perfume manufacture is widespread. In the nineteenth century, advances in chemistry conflicted with the popular view that reproducing the patiently developed harmonies of nature was rather arrogant. Yet while the names of Perkin, Tiemann, Baur, Darzens, Ruzicka, Blanc and Bouveault have today been largely forgotten, it is to these men that modern perfumes owe their existence. Before the chemistry of fragrance established itself, perfumes were composed of high-quality, natural raw materials which amounted to perfumes in themselves. Blenders mixed in a simple way, according to their own creative impulse. The market for fragrances produced in this way was limited by their cost, and, with the exception of eaux de Cologne and some other extracts, perfume remained a luxury reserved for the privileged classes.

From 1830 onwards, some chemists who were not involved in perfume-making undertook research into natural fragrances, initially isolating what seemed the most interesting elements in the essential oils derived from plants. So it was that geraniol, which has the scent of roses, was extracted from essence of citronella using the method of fractional distillation and that menthol was produced by crystallization of essence of mint. These substances were called isolates. After reaching this first stage, scientists were obliged to observe that many of the aromatic components of natural materials could not be isolated, either because they were present in only minute quantities or because separating them would have been too costly, as in the case of the vanillin content of vanilla. Through the process of synthesis, chemists reproduced these substances using elements extracted from other plant essences. The isolation of terpene in essence of pine, for example, yielded terpineol, which is used in lilac blends.

These results encouraged scientists to attempt to recreate such substances using fossil materials, such as oil and coal, rather than plants. They achieved this through synthesis: phenyl ethyl alcohol, a derivative of benzene, replicates the subtle fragrance of roses; benzyl acetate, derived from toluene, has the scent of jasmine; and salicylic acid was used to synthesize coumarin, a new substance which paved the way for the fern group of perfumes. Not content with simply reproducing molecules identical to those in nature, chemists went on to invent artificial fragrant molecules, much to the delight of perfume-makers. This led to a real revolution, in much the same way as the invention of new colors would have radically changed a painter's life: heliotropin became an important element in all Oriental compositions; vanillin helped Guerlain create his finest perfumes; with its scents of leather and smoke, quinoline provided the inspiration for Chanel's *Cuir de Russie*; the warm and long-lasting accents of synthetic musks were used as base notes in compositions where they made excellent fixatives; and ionone was used to reproduce the scent of violets. Lastly, the reduction of fatty acids yielded aldehydes, whose forceful and sometimes nauseating smell initially discouraged their use in perfume manufacture. It was Coco Chanel and her "nose," Ernest Beaux, who first dared to use them in their legendary *No.5*. Although some claim that Ernest Beaux was unwittingly heavy-handed in his use of aldehydes and that this famous perfume was created by accident, the successful result was a family of fragrances that is sure to last as long as perfumery itself.

Since the end of the Second World War, chromatography – a process which identifies the component molecules of a fragrant compound in their various proportions – has offered fascinating possibilities for research of molecules present in only minute traces in natural raw materials. Scientists continued to create marvellous new products, such as the hedione pivotal to Dior's *Eau Sauvage* mentioned earlier, as well as the damascones at the heart of *Les Jardins de Bagatelle* by Guerlain and *Paris* by Yves Saint Laurent. Researchers have benefited more recently from the "headspace" technique, which allows them to capture a flower, a tree or a fragrant atmosphere *in situ* and obtain a kind of genetic fingerprint by identifying their component molecules. This technique is particularly useful for flowers not yet employed in perfumery, such as orchids and wisteria, and also for atmospheric perfumes, such as the smell of the forest floor or the fragrance of the seashore. It also makes for the closest approximation of naturally occurring scents at all stages of their development, something which is not always the case with essential oils and absolute essences, whose fragrance often differs from the smell of a plant in its natural state.

In 1952, the great perfume-blender Ernest Beaux claimed that "We must rely on chemistry to discover the elements from which new and original notes can bloom. There is no doubt that the future of perfume is in the hands of the chemists." More than forty years later, these words still ring true. Science works in tandem with perfumery not by rejecting nature, but by skillfully allying itself with it.

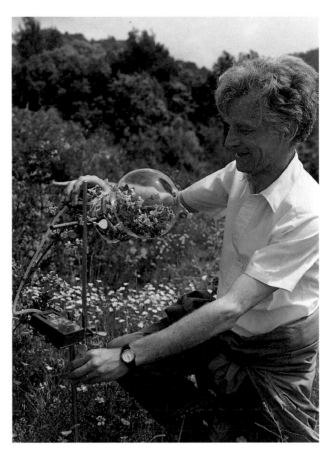

49

The most recent revolution in perfumery has been initiated by the headspace technique, which provides a new source of inspiration to perfume-makers in search of original blends. "Living" perfumes – in this case, those of flowers – are trapped in a glass vessel linked to a machine that analyzes their molecular structure.

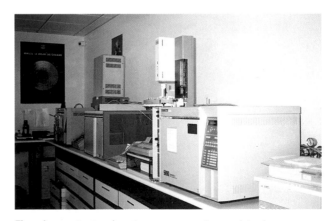

The chromatograph acts as a computer-assisted "fragrance filter," providing the blender with the exact proportion of each chemical component in a perfume. The elusive qualities captured by our sense of smell are thus translated into as many pixels on the screen as there are molecules in a fragrance.

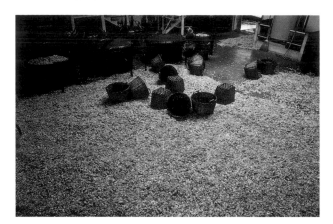

The process begins with the arrival of sack-loads of thousands of flowers.

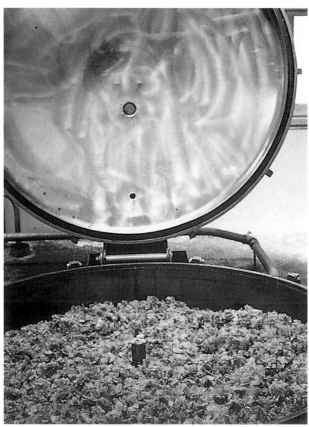

The flowers are then spread out over the floor in cool, dark rooms before being taken to the vats for treatment – steam distillation or, as in this photo, extraction by volatile solvents.

MANUFACTURING PROCESSES

Although the Egyptians had discovered in very early times that certain woods and resins would give off subtle perfumes when burned, many centuries elapsed before methods of transforming flowers, fruits and plants into essences, absolutes and resinoids were discovered. These products are the result of a high level of technical expertise, acquired through experimentation and the constant refinement of the tools involved. Many different machines have to be tested before a final version reaches the modern distillery or extraction workshop.

MACERATION

This is undoubtedly one of the oldest techniques of extraction. Having observed the affinity between fragrant substances and fat, early perfume-makers decided to macerate flowers in fats or oils, which were heated either naturally by the sun or in a bain-marie. Once the absorbent substance was saturated with perfume, it was filtered through material, initially linen and later cotton, to obtain a kind of fragrant ointment. Animal fats and then petroleum jelly were gradually replaced by oils; resins, spices and a few drops of perfumed essences were added to enrich these fragrant pomades.

Advances in distillation and extraction techniques led perfume-makers to rinse the pomades in pure alcohol, which they discovered could absorb their fragrance. In an operation repeated two or three times, the mixture was stirred mechanically and then left to stand before the alcohol and fat were drawn off separately. The alcohol thus became a perfumed extract and was filtered one last time to eliminate all traces of fat.

ENFLEURAGE

Based on the same principle as maceration – the affinity between fragrance and fats – and differing only in that no heat is used, the enfleurage technique has the advantage of being suitable for treating fragile flowers, such as jasmine or tuberose. Before distillation and extraction became common practice, this was the best method of obtaining a fragrance resembling that of the flower.

Rather than being immersed in a hot solution, the petals in this case are placed on a thin layer of fat spread over a sheet of glass, which is supported by a wooden chassis between fifteen and twenty-four inches square. The substance used is a mixture of refined pork and beef fat, stabilized with benzoin. The flowers, which remain alive for a while after picking, are left in the machine for varying lengths of time (twenty-four hours for jasmine, seventy-two for tuberose), removed and then replaced with fresh flowers until the fat is saturated with perfume. In order to dissolve the fragrance, the fat is rinsed in cold alcohol, which is subsequently evaporated to obtain a pomade absolute.

Although today enfleurage is a technique used only by a select few in and around Grasse, it provided employment for large numbers of women in the early years of this century. There were ten or so workers for every hundred chassis and some companies in Grasse had as many as eighty thousand chassis. As soon as they arrived at the factory, the flowers were sorted to remove those which were damp or spoiled. The fat had to be made ready with a wooden comb before they were laid out on it, both to ensure a better distribution of flowers and to aerate the fat so that it absorbed the perfume evenly. Two days later, the défleurage process took place, where the frames were banged on a table to remove the petals. It was estimated that one pound of fat could absorb about three pounds of flowers, but the cost of this lavish technique was extremely high and today it is, understandably, only used for a few exceptional perfumes.

DISTILLATION

This extraction process, radically different from maceration and enfleurage, is based on the principle of the evaporation and subsequent condensation of liquids and relies on the ability of water vapor to carry essential oils. The device used for this technique is the still, whose invention is credited to the Arabs some time between the eighth and tenth centuries. However, the principle of distillation was also familiar to the Greeks and the Egyptians from the fourth or third century BC onwards.

Although at one time it resembled the device used by home-brewers, the still employed in modern perfumery has three parts: the still itself, an oval-shaped vat on top of which is the head, also called the swan neck, which is linked to the condenser, a metal coil situated inside a vat filled with cold water. The product to be distilled (whether it be flowers, herbs, leaves, branches, roots or mosses) is loaded into the vat on perforated shelves, and the water in the bain-marie, located in the false bottom of the vat, is brought to boiling point. Laden with the plant's fragrant molecules, the vapor escapes via the swan neck and then proceeds to the condenser, where it becomes a liquid and falls into the collecting flask, otherwise known as a Florentine vase. Here, the elements separate from each other because of their different densities. The water is generally heavier and remains at the bottom of the flask, while the essential oils, which are not water-soluble, rise to the surface and are siphoned off.

In a number of instances – as is the case with rose water and the orange flower water obtained from orange blossoms – the water produced by distillation is also imbued with essence and is collected to be sold on its own, in this pure form.

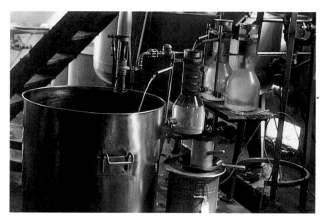

At the end of the distillation process, a plant's essential oil is collected in a flask known as a Florentine vase.

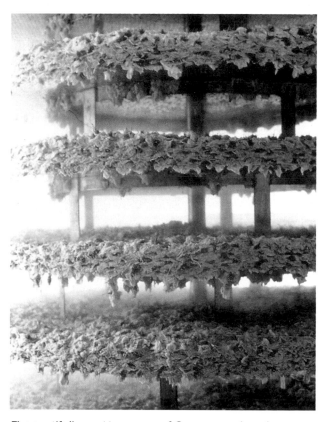

The centifolia, *or May, roses of Grasse are placed on perforated shelves before undergoing extraction by volatile solvents.*

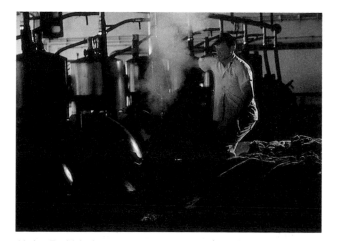

Here, Turkish damascena *roses are treated by steam distillation.*

51

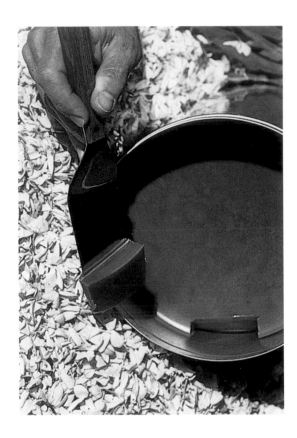

After the solvent has absorbed the perfume, it is evaporated off, leaving a dense paste of varying hardness called a concrete.

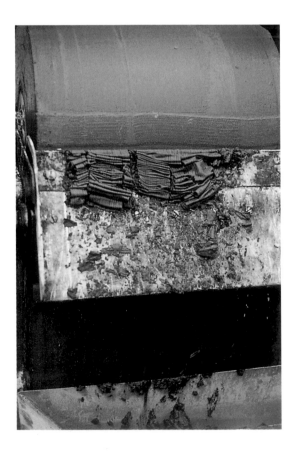

Floral concretes often have a thick consistency, containing waxes and paraffins which are insoluble in alcohol and therefore removed.

The stills used by our ancestors were placed directly onto large stones and heated by fires which had to be kept at as regular a temperature as possible. Since then, techniques have improved and today's stills are driven by low pressure steam, which is, more often than not, generated externally. In this way, the ideal temperature for distillation can be reached and maintained throughout the operation. The days when bizarre tubular contraptions on wheels could be seen in the lavender fields of Provence, distilling the flowers as soon as they were picked, are therefore over. Modern stills, less charming but much more productive, now await the delivery of plants by the truck-load at the distillery.

EXTRACTION BY VOLATILE SOLVENTS

While distillation is very effective with a flower like lavender, or with orris, vetiver, sandalwood, geranium leaves and so on, the results are not always as favorable with other plants. Either the yield of essential oil is very low, or the end product is too far removed from the true scent of the plant. To solve this problem and to be able to treat flowers like the *centifolia* rose, the narcissus or the mimosa, experts perfected a technique whose principle is based on exploiting the affinity of certain solvents with the perfumes contained in fragrant raw materials. From the eighteenth century onwards, scientists had been trying to turn this theory into practice using ether, but production costs were huge and there was the constant danger that the solvents would ignite or explode. Advances in the scientific study of hydrocarbons, coupled with better safety regulations, led to the use of higher quality solvents, mainly hexane and benzene, chosen for their great properties of solubilization and their volatility, which made them easy to evaporate.

Extraction takes place in three thousand litre (780 gallon), stainless steel vats which are filled with perforated trays stacked one on top of the other so that the plants are not packed down and crushed, thus allowing the solvent to circulate freely. Machines with rotating drums which make the continuous treatment of plants possible are also used. After the extractor is loaded, the solvents are introduced via a system of sluices. The plants are then stripped of their perfume by successive solvent rinses – the appropriate length of contact depends on the nature of the plant and the particular solvent used. Once saturated with fragrance, the solvent is first decanted to remove excess moisture and then transferred to a vacuum still, where partial distillation takes place. It is evaporated, retrieved and then recycled in various successive processes, leaving a paste-like mixture, composed of fragrant molecules, waxes and pigments, at the bottom of the machine. This mixture, when the result of the treatment of dry plants (like roots, seeds, mosses, balsam, gums or resins) is called a resinoid; it is called a concrete when obtained specifically from the treatment of flowers. While perfume-makers generally use resinoids in their compositions just as they are, concretes are subject to further refinement. Floral concretes often have a thick consistency, containing waxes and paraffins that are insoluble in alcohol. Therefore, once the waxes are initially filtered out, the concrete rinsed repeatedly in alcohol in machines called *batteuses* to dissolve the fragrant molecules. As waxes congeal at low temperatures, the concrete-alcohol mixture is subsequently frozen to between -12°C (10°F) and -15°C (5°F) and filtered again to remove permanently all traces of wax. Finally, the mixture undergoes low pressure distillation and evaporation of the alcohol yields an absolute essence, known in the profession simply as an absolute.

EXPRESSION

This process is used by perfume-makers solely for extraction of the citrus oils from fruits such as oranges, lemons and mandarins. The essential oils of these fruits are contained in tiny glands in the zest. When peeling a citrus fruit, a spray of little droplets is evident; these droplets of liquid are a mixture of fragrant essence and water. This same principle of extraction is applied to perfume manufacture. Today the essence is drawn out by sophisticated pieces of machinery, but before mechanization, the job was done by hand. In Sicily and Calabria, for example, bergamot and lemon were treated using a leather glove studded with small pieces of pumice stone. The workers scraped the fruit with one hand and collected the essential oil in the other with a sponge, which they then squeezed out into a bucket. Obviously, this method, known as *a la spugna*, produced a much lower yield than today's machines and cost a great deal more in labor.

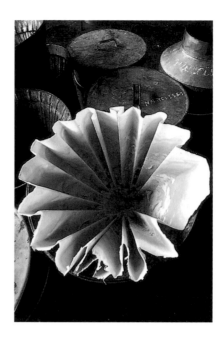

For a purer result, the concrete-alcohol mixture is rinsed several times in alcohol and then frozen to filter out the waxes. The alcohol is subsequently evaporated off, yielding a product coveted by all perfume-makers – the absolute.

53

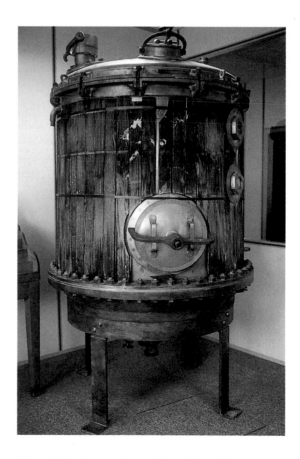

The still is a descendant of the alchemist's retort and, before the invention of modern machinery, perfumes were refined in stills like this one.

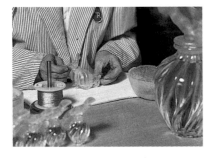

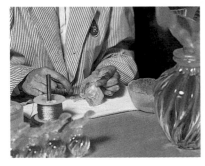

BLENDING, MACERATION AND PACKAGING

Essential oils, absolute essences and resinoids are produced by raw materials processing companies, often based in Grasse, which usually undertake extraction and distillation in their own factories there. There are, however, some raw materials so delicate – as is often the case with exotic or rare flowers – that they are bought directly from their country of origin in a ready-processed state. What also frequently happens is that a raw material is treated in the place where it is grown and then transported as a concrete to Grasse, where it is subsequently turned into an absolute. Perfume-makers, particularly the major names, buy from either these local processing companies or else directly from the producers. Some of the major names, however, do their own blending of both natural and synthetic raw materials. These are carefully weighed out according to the secret in-house formula created by the elected "nose," producing what is called a concentrate. This is true of Jean Patou, for example, whose house perfume-blender Jean Kerléo buys and checks in person all the raw materials which have been brought in, and supervises the production of every bottle of perfume as it leaves the factory at Levallois-Perret, near Paris, for world-wide distribution. Other perfume-makers have their raw materials sent to reputed perfume-blending companies, who know the formula and are therefore able to produce the concentrate. These concentrates are then transported either to the factories which are owned and run by the major names to companies which specialize in packaging and undertake work for numerous different brands.

The next stage of production is called maceration and involves leaving the concentrate in contact with alcohol in huge stainless steel vats for a prolonged period of time in order to obtain an optimum quality of perfume. The quantity of alcohol used depends on the type of product required: extract, also called perfume; eau de toilette; eau de parfum, otherwise known as parfum de toilette; eau de Cologne and so on. An extract usually contains between 15 and 20% perfume concentrate dissolved in the alcohol and eau de toilette between 5 and 10%, whereas the

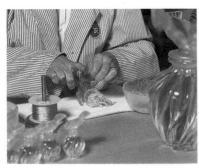

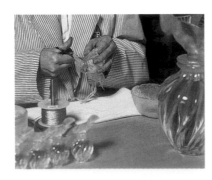

Baudruchage – *one of the most prestigious jobs in the packaging department. Using a highly skilful technique, a moistened piece of leather is placed on top of each stopper and then tied with gold thread, thus guaranteeing an unadulterated product to the consumer.*

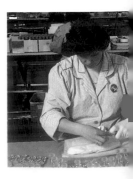

proportion in eau de parfum, which is halfway between the two, differs according to the brand.

In France, the alcohol normally used is derived from beetroot and refined so as to have a neutral smell. The length of maceration depends on the type of product and can vary from a few weeks to three months, during which time a precipitate of plant substances is formed. This deposit is removed by a technique called *glaçage* (or solidification) at temperatures between 0°C (32°F) and -10°C (14°F), followed by filtration, thus producing a transparent liquid. The vats are thoroughly rinsed after each subsequent maceration, and, in the case of great perfumes, the same vats must be used for the same blend.

Once the contents have been prepared, all that remains is for the bottles to be filled and then packaged. In modern factories, the maceration vats are often linked by a myriad of pipes to the automated packing machines, situated on the floor above, which fill a regular stream of bottles on a conveyor belt. A long bottling process takes place: quality control, decoration, the addition of a batch number to each bottle which guarantees its authenticity, the fitting of the stopper, labeling and so on. The bottles are then conveyed by the box-load to the packaging section. Here, dozens of workers at long tables check each one individually, rejecting any which are flawed, then wiping the bottles one by one as well as ensuring, where necessary, that the atomizer is working properly. Bottles of perfume extract undergo a further process, called *baudruchage*, where the stopper is covered with a small cap of leather (traditionally a piece of bull's intestine, previously soaked in a bowl of water), which is then tied with gold thread. This technique is the sole preserve of the major perfume houses and guarantees to the customer that the product they are buying is unadulterated. Only a few experienced workers are capable of performing this prestigious task which requires skill and painstaking precision. The final stage involves putting the bottle into its box or other container (a toilet kit, for example), which is then wrapped by machine in plastic. Lastly, the bottles are stored on palets in enormous warehouses before being shipped to distributors and perfume shops throughout the world.

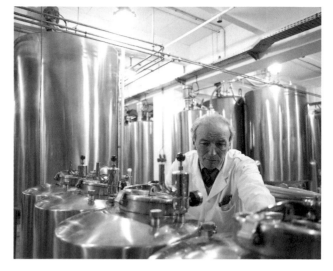

A technician carefully monitors the maceration vats, where the perfume concentrate is mixed with alcohol. It can take as long as three months before the perfume develops its full potential and can then be bottled.

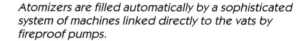

Atomizers are filled automatically by a sophisticated system of machines linked directly to the vats by fireproof pumps.

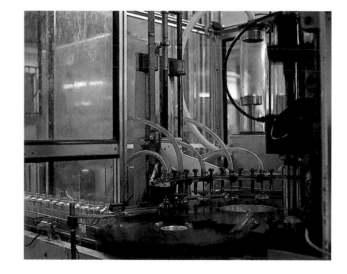

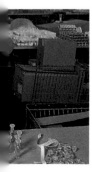
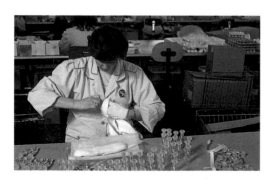
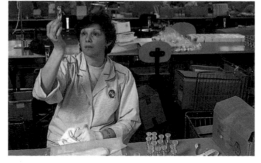

At the Nina Ricci factory in Ury, south of Paris, each atomizer is checked by spraying a few drops of perfume onto absorbent material. The bottles are then wiped and their clarity checked before packaging.

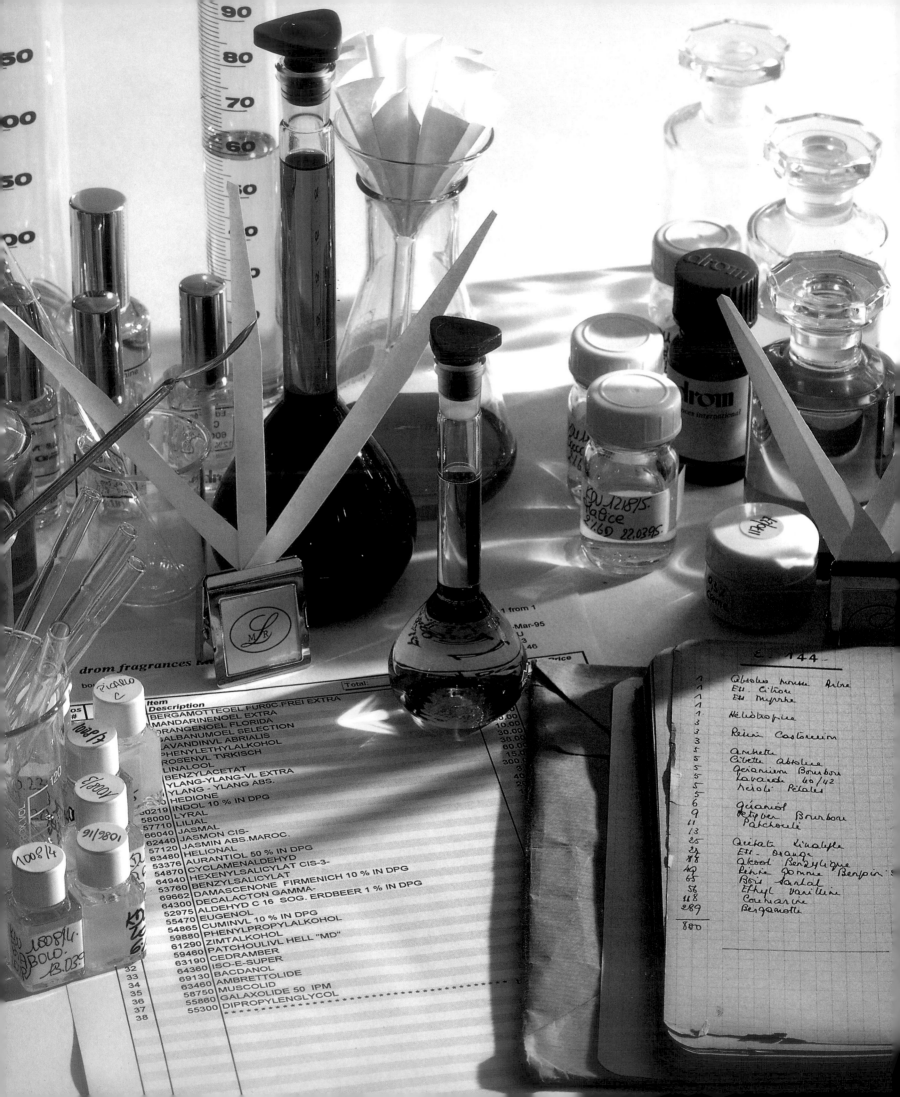

THE ART OF PERFUME MAKING

A perfume is a work of art born of its blender's memory, discernment and skill. Referred to in the trade as "noses," these artists use more than just their sense of smell in the creation of their fragrant works of art. In the same way that a musician must learn the rudiments of music before being able to sight-read or compose a score, perfume-makers unanimously agree that they draw first on their memory and the hundreds of smells carefully recorded in it.

While in the early years of this century all the major perfume-makers and couturiers employed their own in-house blender, the situation today is entirely different. There are only three of the great perfume houses left which retain such a privilege: Chanel, Guerlain and Jean Patou. The majority of perfume-makers now resort to blending companies, whose elected "noses" produce perfumes for the big names. They must of course adhere strictly to their clients' very specific requirements.

Perfumery is a luxury industry which has now become subject to very strict regulation (particularly with regard to international legislation governing the use of ingredients) as well as economic constraints. Publicity and market research play a prominent part in the launch of any new perfume – ample evidence of which is provided by the evolution of advertising material.

In order to help blenders in their job, perfumes are classified into families, thereby establishing a language of common reference. As perfumery is not an exact science, and there are as many different interpretations of a smell as there are individuals, the family names have been chosen to reflect characteristic sense impressions created by the member perfumes. In France, the technical division of the Société des Parfumeurs has produced a universal system of classification comprising seven families, which lists all existing perfumes whose composition is known. During the course of the following pages, you will doubtless recognize your favorite perfume and hopefully discover something new about how it is produced and perhaps the key to why you like it.

While computer databases may today have replaced the hand-written notebook as a means of storing precious perfume formulas, the basic tools used by the "noses" remain the same – test strips, pipettes, test tubes and so on.

THE NOSE

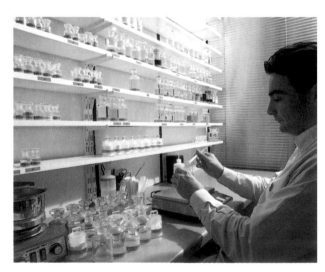

"Noses" once used essences and absolutes kept in huge flasks wrapped in leather to protect them from the light. The bottles illustrated were used in the last century by perfume-blenders at Guerlain.

Today, blenders entrust their formula to an assistant who weighs out a perfume's ingredients. Using a bain-marie, these are then heated in a container fitted with a mixer to produce a homogenous blend.

The artists who fuse the magic of the plant world with the techniques of chemistry are known by many different names – perfume-blender, perfume-creator, perfumer, "nose" and so on – but who are these men and women involved in this fascinating profession and what distinguishes them from us?

There was a time when the job of perfume-maker was handed down from father to son and success depended almost entirely on being a native of Grasse. Fortunately, with the establishment of a number of specialist training schools, membership of the profession has gradually become less restricted. While this apprenticeship involves committing to memory and understanding how both natural and synthetic raw materials can be used, the majority of "noses" enter the profession by working as assistants to perfume-blenders before becoming blenders themselves. When asked what particular skills are required to succeed in the job, the "noses" all give more or less the same answer: simply a normal sense of smell and an interest in perfumery. When pressed, they will add that a lengthy training period and an excellent memory are also required. However, these answers show signs of excessive modesty, for blending a perfume is also an artistic process. It is vital that the "noses" use their imagination and discernment to create a fragrance. As Jean Kerléo, perfume-blender at Jean Patou, explains, "A perfume is inspired by the discovery of new smells and new people." The inspiration for a fragrance therefore comes first from the mind of its creator, not from a series of bottles smelled individually at a desk. "When perfume-makers write a formula, they have quite a good idea of what it will smell like," explains blender Karine Dubreuil. Only after it has been committed to paper will a perfume take "physical" shape, with the weighing and blending of its constituent raw materials. Here begins a long series of experiments, for the first blend is rarely the one that matches the perfume-maker's mental picture perfectly.

Like other artists, perfume-blenders often have difficulty in knowing when to stop. "My initial ideas are often the best ones", admits Françoise Caron. "I believe that the addition or removal of ingredients will not improve my blend to any significant degree. Some blenders are real perfectionists and can spend months refining their perfume." Today, the creation of a perfume is above all a team effort. The majority of "noses" work for perfume-blending companies, inventing fragrances to the specification of their clients – couturiers, jewelers, designers, perfume houses, etc. These various companies share the world market and usually compete with one another in the creation of the same perfume; while only three major French perfume-makers – Chanel, Guerlain and Jean Patou – have their own in-house blender. Whatever the circumstances, the "noses" must work in tandem with the marketing department. The marketing experts are responsible for the "initial brief" which is the basis for any perfume launched on today's market. It generally takes the form of a synopsis, sometimes accompanied by a photograph or video, describing the target market, sex, age, social category and personality of its wearer, the family of fragrances to which it will belong, references to known perfumes, etc. Once familiar with the brief, the blenders set to work. While they are required to create something original, they will already have ideas in reserve, in much the same way as a painter makes sketches before starting work on a canvas. According to Olivier Cresp, creator of Thierry Mugler's *Angel*, a specific brief does not necessarily exclude innovation: "The spirit of adventure of major couturiers such as Mugler, Gaultier and Miyake benefits us all, allowing us to be daring and innovative. The note of confectionery in *Angel* could never have been used with a classic couturier." Thierry Mugler had asked him to create a perfume reminiscent of his childhood, evoking fairground smells of hot nougat, candy floss, toasted hazelnuts and chocolate.

Between five and ten companies are usually consulted for the launch of a single perfume, but only one will win the contract. It takes about eighteen months from the delivery of the brief to the client's final decision, and a further year before the fragrance is launched. There is often a great deal of frustration involved in the process. The client is in a position to impose his demands and change a formula judged successful by its blender. Some briefs have taken over eight years to reach completion. When legislation makes it impossible to use a particular ingredient, blenders have even been asked to re-design an existing perfume. This happened with bergamot, which can only be used in very low concentration, and musk ambrette, which is now banned. Both were once found in two famous perfumes, the formulas for which had to be rewritten. Here, the research department comes into its own, working on the development of new molecules for the blenders to assess. This need for teamwork and the all-pervading influence of the marketing department might be seen as a limitation. However, many blenders would agree with the words of Jacques Polge, chief perfume-maker at Chanel: "Solitude is dangerous. You risk making an innovation that nobody will understand. As Goethe said 'Create a better future by developing elements of the past.'"

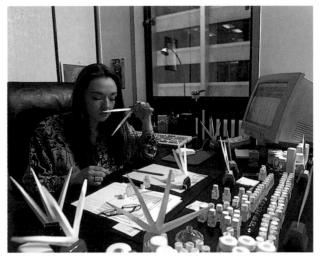

Karine Dubreuil, perfume-blender with the DROM blending company: "For me, a great perfume is the product of a simple composition in a major key, with a clear main theme and a strong, unmistakable personality."

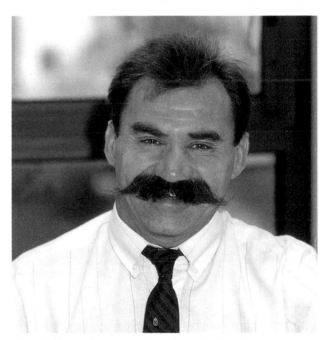

Maurice Roucel, perfume-blender with the Quest company – creator of Tocade *by Rochas and* 24, Faubourg *by Hermès.*

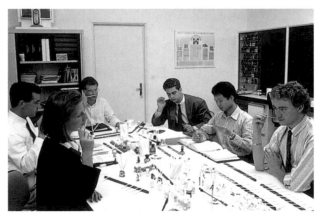

The three-year training course at the Roure-Givaudan school enables two or three young perfume-blenders to work with a "nose" after eighteen months of tutorials.

59

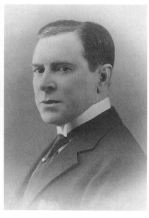

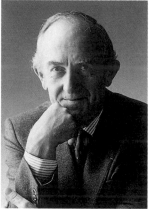

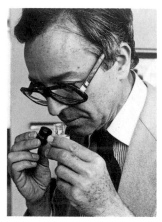

Left: *Germaine Cellier was the first woman to join the elite rank of perfume-blenders. Her prolific imagination and independent spirit have left their mark on this marvellous profession.*
Right: *At the same time, perfume-maker and businessman François Coty was the creator of* Chypre, *which established an eponymous family of perfumes.*

Left: *Nicolas Mamounas, the creator of numerous perfumes for Rochas.*
Right: *Jean Kerléo is in charge of perfumes at Jean Patou and is also an eminent member of the Société Française des Parfumeurs.*

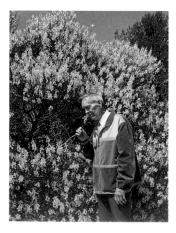

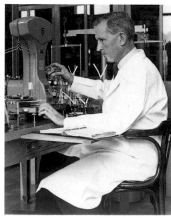

Left: *Edmond Roudnitska, one of the most famous "noses" of modern times, whose most notable creations include* Femme *by Rochas,* Eau d'Hermès *and especially Christian Dior's* Eau Sauvage.
Right: *The name of André Fraysse is invariably associated with Lanvin, for whom he created some superb compositions.*

FAMOUS PERFUME BLENDERS

When glove and perfume-makers, apothecaries and chemists blended fragrances in the back of their shops, their reputations rarely spread beyond a group of regular customers. Their skills were regarded as those of a competent craftsman and their clients generally considered them to be mere purveyors of scent. With the dawn of industrialization, the wider availability of perfumes led to an increase in their creators' power and prestige, elevating a few names from the anonymity of the craftsman to the rank of artist and entrepreneur.

The house of Guerlain, founded in 1828 by Pierre-François-Pascal Guerlain, symbolizes this progression. Perfume-maker by appointment to the Empress Eugénie, Guerlain acquired a reputation which led his son Aimé to create *Jicky* and, from 1892 onwards, his grandson Jacques to produce the most innovative perfumes of the day including *Mitsouko, Shalimar, L'Heure Bleue, Vol de Nuit* and *Après l'Ondée.* Jean-Paul Guerlain, the current "nose," represents the fifth generation of perfume-makers to have followed in the family tradition.

Born in 1874, the same year as Jacques Guerlain, François Coty was one of a new breed of artist-cum-businessman. He initially sold his perfumes through large department stores, but later opened his own shop on the Place Vendôme in Paris, establishing a fruitful partnership with the glass-maker Lalique until the Wall Street Crash of 1929 abruptly halted the expansion of his business. Apart from *L'Origan* and *Émeraude,* his most famous creation was *Chypre,* whose blend of base notes was so original that it founded a family of perfumes.

The name of Ernest Beaux is linked with the most famous of all perfumes – *Chanel No.5.* Born in Moscow in 1881, he soon made a name for himself at Rallet, a Russian perfume-maker of French extraction. After being mobilized to France during the war, he resumed his career in Grasse, and in 1920 produced two series of tests numbered 1 to 5 and 20 to 24 for Coco Chanel. Original for being the first perfume to use aldehydes, strong-smelling synthetic products, it was number 5 that caught the couturière's attention. Ernest Beaux also created *No.22* and *Cuir de Russie* for Chanel, as well as *Soir de Paris* for Bourjois.

Born in Bordeaux in 1909, Germaine Cellier began studying chemistry in Paris in 1930 and became the first woman to enter the enclave of perfume-blenders. She joined the Roure-Bertrand-Dupont perfumery company, where she soon made a name for herself. At that time, Roure, which produced the raw materials sold to perfume-makers, decided to expand into creating ready-made perfumes on its own and persuade couturiers to launch them under their own name. These were the ideal conditions for Germaine Cellier to give free rein to her imagination. She liked brief, simple formulas, making her perfumes daring, straightforward and a little stark. She was convinced that perfume-blending was a gift, which had no rules and could not be learned. In 1944, she created the superb *Bandit,* a sensual and animal chypre fragrance with a note of leather, for the designer Robert Piguet. Her collaboration with the couturier Pierre Balmain produced *Vent Vert*, the first perfume with a green note and whose formula included a bold 8% concentration of galbanum. Her fiery temperament and passionate stands on matters of perfume composition distanced her from Roure, and in 1946 she became the managing director of the Exarome company, where the first perfume advertisement was filmed. In that same year she created Nina Ricci's first perfume *Cœur Joie*, a beautiful floral aldehyde. Numerous equally original fragrances followed: *Jolie Madame* for Balmain (1953), *Monsieur Balmain* (1964) and several Elizabeth Arden perfumes for the American market.

It is interesting to note the loyalty that is forged between a perfume-maker and a couturier once their first perfume has been launched, as in the case of André Fraysse and Jeanne Lanvin. Their first creation was *My Sin* (1925), followed by *Arpège* (1927), a subtle blend of Bulgarian rose, jasmine, mock orange, lily of the valley and honeysuckle, contained in the famous black sphere which was to become the bottle for all Lanvin perfumes. "Perfume, like love, must captivate a woman immediately," claimed Fraysse, who also produced *Scandal* (1932), *Rumeur* (1932) and *Prétexte* (1937).

While these names are known to the profession and a few well-informed outsiders, perfumery is undoubtedly the only art of the twentieth century that keeps the majority of its practitioners anonymous. The opportunity must be taken to acknowledge the following talents: Henri Almeras, creator of Jean Patou's *Joy* and most of the Parfums de Rosine; Louis Armingeat, creator of the majority of L.T.Piver's perfumes; Maurice Blanchet (*Je Reviens* and *Sans Adieu* for Worth); Jean Carles (*Tabu* and *Canoé* for Dana, *Ma Griffe* for Carven); Ernest Daltroff (*Narcisse Noir* and *Fleurs de Rocaille* for Caron); and Henri Robert (*Pour Monsieur* and *No.19* for Chanel). Perhaps the best definition of perfume was expressed by Edmond Roudnitska, one of the greatest contemporary perfume-blenders and author of many reference works on the subject: "A beautiful perfume is one which causes a 'shock,' a sensory shock which at first acquaintance jolts the spirit, followed by a psychological shock which lasts all the longer for the perfume slowly taking shape ... Perfume is an act of poetic thought."

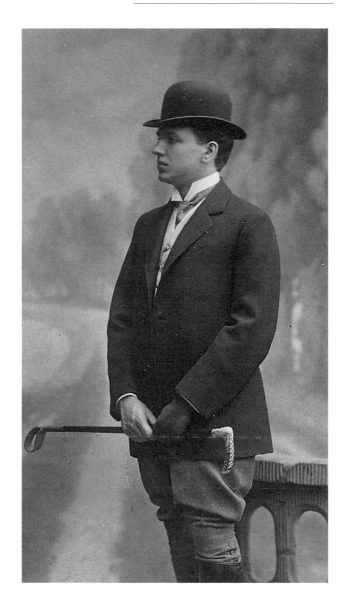

61

Ernest Beaux – a young man with the air of a dandy who was the inspired creator of the world-famous Chanel No.5, *as well as* Soir de Paris *by Bourjois. The use of synthetic raw materials in his innovative compositions contributed to the advancement of perfumery.*

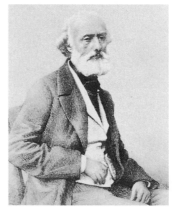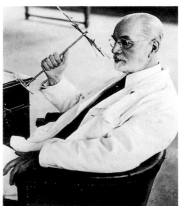

At Guerlain, the profession of perfume-blender has been handed down from one generation to the next. For over a century, this great family has been creating superb compositions whose style is so immediately recognizable that the word 'guerlinade' has been coined to describe it.

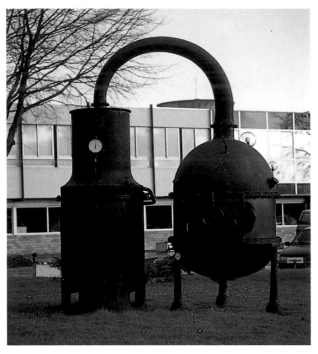

Above: *Modern distillation procedures have seen the development of highly sophisticated pieces of machinery like this turbo-still.*

Below: *The era of the stills used by early perfume-makers is well and truly over.*

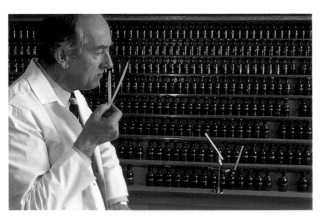

Jean Kerléo, perfume-blender at Jean Patou. Test strips are an indispensable tool for the "nose" – once sprayed with a few drops of a raw material or a composition, they enable him to assess the quality of a perfume and to examine its development.

GLOSSARY OF PERFUME

Words followed by an asterisk are defined elsewhere in the glossary.

Absolute: Absolute essences are obtained from either concretes* or resinoids*, which are rinsed several times in alcohol. In order to remove any waxes, the alcoholic solution is frozen and then filtered, before undergoing low pressure distillation* to expel the alcohol, thus concentrating the mixture.

Base: 1. Word used to describe the characteristically plain-smelling composition* which results from the mixture of several different raw materials. It is a ready-made element, used by a "nose"* as an individual raw material. 2. The base note contains the least volatile constituents of a perfume and is its most persistent element, remaining after the top* and middle* notes have evaporated.

Blend: Effect obtained by mixing together two or three raw materials, or plain notes*. A blend is described as harmonious when the proportions and fragrant intensity of its ingredients are in equal balance.

Chromatography: Scientific process which identifies and analyzes the molecular components of products used in perfumery.

Composition: Final mixture of a selection of both natural and synthetic products and bases*. Perfume-makers use the term to describe the product obtained at the end of the blending process.

Concentrate: Term used to describe a composition* once it has been blended according to the specific proportions of the "nose's"* formula. Concentrates are then diluted in alcohol in percentages which vary depending on the type of product required – whether it be an extract*, eau de parfum, eau de toilette, etc.

Concrete: Solid or semi-solid substance obtained by the extraction of the fragrant constituents of certain plants (such as jasmine, rose or narcissus) using volatile solvents (such as hexane or benzene).

Diffusion: The way in which a smell develops when it is exposed to the air.

Distillation: Steam treatment of the fragrant elements contained in certain natural raw materials, transforming them into essential oils*.

Dominant: Word used to describe the most pronounced fragrant note* in a composition*, e.g. a floral note with a dominant of jasmine.

Essence: see Essential oil.

Essential oil (or Essence): Term applied to the volatile aromatic products extracted from plants by either distillation* or expression*, such as essence of rose, sandalwood or lemon.

Expression: Technique employed to extract certain essential oils*, mainly from the zest of citrus fruits, using machine presses, centrifuges, etc.

Extract: see Perfume.

Fragrance: Word derived from Latin, used to describe the agreeable scent of a perfume, whereas the word "smell" can also refer to something unpleasant.

Headspace: Recently introduced technique for analyzing the volatile constituents of fragrant materials in a vacuum.

Infuse: Verb used in perfumery to describe the absorption of the soluble elements of a solid by a liquid during prolonged exposure to each other – sometimes several years. Musk, ambergris and oak moss are treated in this way.

Jus: Term commonly applied in the perfume industry to the alcoholic solution of a perfume concentrate*.

Line: Range of products derived from a single fragrance* and marketed under the same name.

Middle: The middle note, or modifier, determines the character of a perfume and is the stage in its development after the top* note has faded and before the base* note evolves.

Nose: Word which, as well as referring to the olfactory organ, is the name given in the industry to the people who create perfumes.

Note: Characteristic fragrance* of a raw material or a composition*, e.g. a floral, green or spicy note.

Organ: Musical analogy employed by perfume-makers to describe the extensive variety of raw materials and bases at their disposal. The words "keyboard" and "palette" are also used.

Perfume: The most concentrated, and usually most costly, product in a given line*, also known as an extract. Often used incorrectly as a synonym of fragrance* or note*, the word also refers to the finished product of a perfume-maker's work.

Preservative: Chemical agent sometimes added by perfume-makers to their compositions* to delay the effects of oxidization.

Resinoid: Resinous product obtained by solvent extraction of certain natural balsams, gums and resins, generally used as a base* note.

Smell: Word applied in perfumery specifically to raw materials and plain notes*, as opposed to the word "fragrance"*, which refers to the more complex scent of a blended perfume.

Test-strip: Narrow strip of special glueless and highly absorbent paper – indispensable in perfumery and chemistry – which, when dipped in a composition* or raw material, allows the perfume-maker to smell the product, assess its quality and monitor its development (top*, middle* and base* notes).

Theme: Principal blend around which the "nose"* creates a perfume.

Top: The top note of a perfume is the fragrant impression created when it is first applied to the skin, and is composed of its most volatile* constituents.

Trail: Term used by perfume-makers to refer to the fragrant impressions detected in the air when somebody wearing a perfume passes by.

Turn: A perfume is described as having turned when chemical alterations produced by aging and exposure to air, heat or light have caused a change in its smell and color.

Volatile: Term applied to a scent which evaporates very quickly.

Volume: Term used to describe a perfume's ability to spread over a wide area when in contact with the air.

(Glossary produced using material published by the *Comité français du parfum*.)

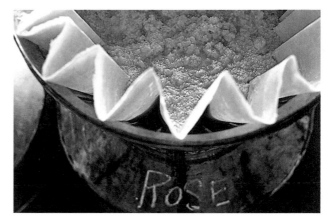

Concrete of rose is obtained by extraction of the fragrant elements of the flower using volatile solvents. This solid or semi solid substance is subsequently transformed into an absolute essence.

63

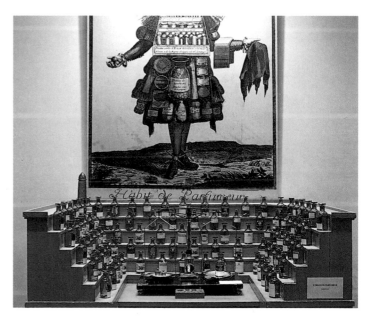

A souvenir from another age, this "perfume organ" was once used by blenders to arrange their raw materials. Today, the tiny bottles are usually kept on shelves and weighed using electronic instruments.

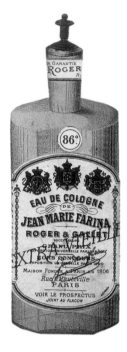

At the end of the last century, perfume-makers began to understand the importance of well-designed labels and packaging for their fragrances. Roger & Gallet, which played a major role in modern perfumery, had a particular talent for packaging.
Left: Rêve Fleuri.
Right: Jean-Marie Farina Eau de Cologne, which Roger & Gallet markets today under the name of Extra-Vieille.

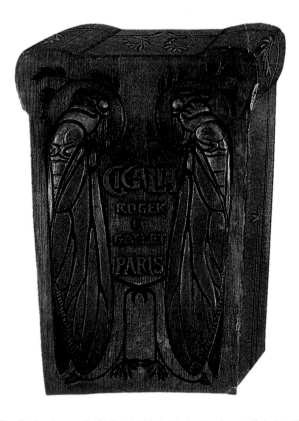

Cigalia by Roger & Gallet (1924). Note the beautiful detail of the box designed to contain the bottle. Made of wood veneer, it features two opposing cicadas with veined wings – the relief is embossed and a bronze patina applied to it, while the graphics are in poker-work.

ADVERTISING AND MARKETING

Using words to evoke a smell is no easy task, and recruiting people capable of persuading others to buy a perfume can be difficult. The fragrance itself only enters the equation at the last minute, when it is bought in a shop. A perfume needs, therefore, to exist in an imaginary visual universe that emphasizes its personality and character.

Perfume's increasing popularity with a wider public at the end of the last century coincided with the beginnings of advertising, but at the time this led to changes in little more than label design or the quality of stoppers and packaging. In those days, the contents of a bottle were its most valuable commercial asset, with the container regarded as a mere necessity. The names of the perfumes themselves provided the clearest guide to their composition – *Jasmin* and *Rose* by Molinard, Houbigant's *Violette Pourpre* and *Fougère Royale*, *Rose Jacqueminot* and *Jasmin de Corse* by Coty – and, predictably, labels were decorated with floral motifs and women at their dressing tables. As the label clearly described each product, sometimes giving directions for use like a medicine, buying a perfume was a straightforward process. Containers came in the standard shapes and sizes sold by any pharmacist, excepting the beautiful and expensive bottles which were bought separately to be filled with a perfume of choice. It is interesting to note the revival of this tradition initiated by Thierry Mugler's *Angel,* whose beautiful star-shaped bottle can be refilled (though no mention is made of perhaps refilling it with a different perfume).

With the increasingly widespread use of synthetic products and a move away from single-fragrance scents towards blends which were both more sophisticated and less easy to describe, perfumes' names became more lyrical. At the same time, products began to be aimed at specific sections of the market and were given more distinct personalities. Perfumes designed for young girls or women, for day or evening wear, and for summer or winter appeared for the first time – it was even fashionable at one stage to add perfume to furs. Of course, this proliferation of fragrances, each with their own target clientele, brought with it a greater degree of individuality to the names and types of packaging used.

At the 1900 World Fair in Paris, Guerlain launched its latest creation, a perfume whose name was an innocent declaration of love – *Voilà Pourquoi J'Aimais Rosine* (That's Why I Loved Rosine). Its vase-shaped bottle topped with an amazing bouquet of silk begonias mirrored the charming naïvete of the name. The concept of the product as a whole and the consistency of design echoing between the name, the bottle and the perfume itself perhaps make this the first real instance of marketing, as yet an unknown field which was to become perfume's modern means of communication. From 1910 onwards, the vast majority of new perfumes took a similar design approach, where the name and the bottle shape combine to create an imaginary world: *Scarabée* by L.T.Piver with its beetle-shaped bottle; *Nuit de Chine*, in the Parfums de Rosine series, with the Chinese-influenced design of its bottle, box and graphics; the beautiful Lalique bottle for Coty's *Ambre Antique*, which features the silhouette of a woman draped in a toga; *Cigalia* by Roger & Gallet, decorated with two cicadas; and finally Monne's *Rêve sur le Nil* which features a bottle in the shape of a pharaoh's head crowned with a lotus flower stopper.

After periods during which the work of an unrestrained imagination can sometimes stretch the boundaries of good taste, the avant-garde usually returns to a more sober, even austere, style. Thus, just as Le Corbusier and Robert Mallet-Stevens brought the teachings of the Bauhaus to France in the Twenties, radically changing the architectural world through their rejection of decoration and use of light to reveal purity of form, Gabrielle Chanel revolutionized perfumery with *No.5*. Quite apart from its daring use of aldehydes and the choice of the most neutral name possible at a time when perfumes called *Toujours Moi, Nuit de Noël* and *Rêve d'Or* were all the rage, its bottle is the perfect artistic expression of the simple function of a container. This sharp-cornered glass rectangle, with its emerald cut stopper and black graphics emblazoned on a stark white background, is a modern classic which has been exhibited at the New York Museum of Modern Art. Although the company admits to making regular slight revisions to the bottle, its restraint and ease of line have ensured that it remained the world's best-selling perfume throughout this century.

Faced with the astonishing success of Chanel *No.5*, other perfume-makers had no hesitation in borrowing the name directly. With a nerve unimaginable today, Molyneux launched *Le Numéro Cinq*, Alice Choquet then named one of her compositions *Double Cinq* and Henri Bendel took things a stage further by christening a fragrance *Cinque, Triple Cinque*! A vogue for numbers became established, with many perfume-makers using figures (*Le Dix* by Balenciaga, and *1,000* by Jean Patou, for example) which they sometimes attached to the company name (*Givenchy III, Azzaro 9, Scherrer 2, Gucci no.3* and so on). Chanel, for its part, launched *No.22* and later *No.19*.

While Coco Chanel enjoyed great fame in the pre-war fashion world, she nevertheless had a talented rival in the Italian baroness Elsa Schiaparelli. This strong personality quickly won hearts with a style whose originality bordered on eccentricity and which bore clear

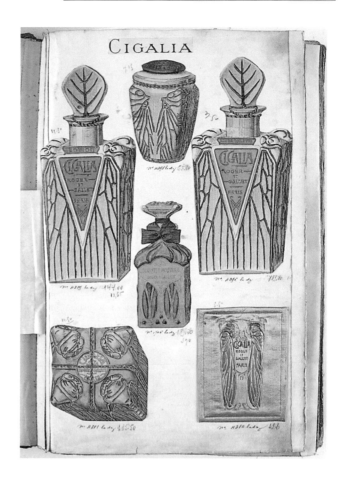

Cigalia, *with a bottle created by René Lalique, was sold from a catalogue by salesmen to individual perfume-sellers. This illustration is taken from a catalogue in use until 1920.*

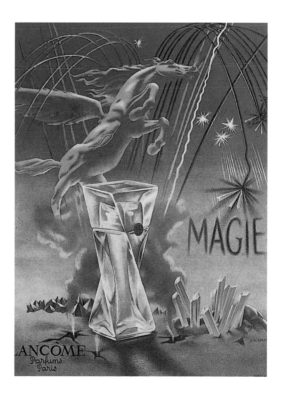

Magie *by Lancôme (1950). Armand Petitjean, Lancôme's founder, considered advertising as prestige weapon for the brand – hence the imagery borrowed from Salvador Dali for this poster designed by Edmond-Marc Pérot.*

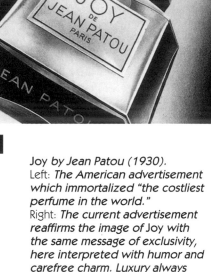

Joy by Jean Patou (1930).
Left: *The American advertisement which immortalized "the costliest perfume in the world."*
Right: *The current advertisement reaffirms the image of* Joy *with the same message of exclusivity, here interpreted with humor and carefree charm. Luxury always sells.*

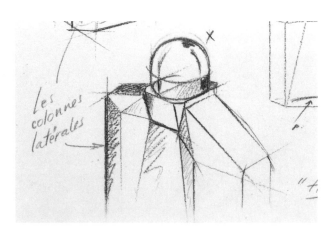

Bottle designers are at the same time artists and technicians who play a pivotal role in a perfume's success by incarnating a dream.

influences from her friends in the Dada and Surrealist movements. Her favorite color was a bright, vivid pink, christened "shocking pink" by her friend the couturier Paul Poiret.

She decided that the names of all her perfumes would begin with an 's,' the initial letter of her surname, and so it was that in 1928 she launched *S*, which failed to attain the success she had hoped for, then in 1933, *Schiap, Salut* and *Soucis*. However, the period from 1936 to 1938 was undoubtedly her most creative. First she produced *Shocking* – its amazing, Surrealist-inspired bottle in the shape of a designer's dummy with the figure of Mae West, one of her clients. It would seem that the actress was something of a muse for perfume-makers, for her curves also inspired the bottle for *Femme,* by her friend Marcel Rochas. The bottle for *Shocking* also features a tape measure hung around its neck and crossed at the waist, as well as a necklace of fabric flowers. The next perfume, *Sleeping,* took the form of a burning candle in a holder, with a red crystal stopper creating the flame and a pale blue, snuffer-shaped box extending the image further. In 1945, Salvador Dali designed the magnificent bottle for *Le Roy Soleil,* whose golden stopper in the shape of a radiant and pensive-looking sun and bottle like a rock, reflecting a blue and gold sea, were kept in a superb shell-shaped box. Unfortunately, the popularity of the Schiaparelli style declined after the War and the company closed down in 1954.

The 's' alliteration was a simple, effective way of creating a family bond between perfumes with varying individual characteristics, as well as providing a signature. This need to underline that different fragrances have been conceived in a similar spirit, along with the habit of launching a new perfume on the back of an existing success, determined the name of many perfumes. At Hermès, *Calèche* in 1961, followed by *Équipage* and *Amazone,* all refer back to the company's original speciality, saddlery. Between 1947 and 1979, Dior lent his surname to a tight cluster of perfumes – *Miss Dior, Diorama, Diorissimo, Diorling, Diorella,* and *Dioressence.* At Jean Patou the effect was less narcissistic. Names were linked to current events : *Normandie* marking the launch of the famous liner in 1935; *Vacances* coinciding with the introduction of holiday pay in France in 1936; *Colony,* produced in 1938 when the clouds of war were gathering and people dreamed of escape; and *L'Heure Attendue,* created in 1946 to commemorate the Liberation.

Today, deciding on a name for a fragrance is a long and complicated process. In what is now a global market, the first hurdle involves finding a name which can be easily pronounced in all major languages without having awkward meanings in any of them. Bearing in mind that computers are working non-stop to produce a pleasant-sounding name which companies can register all over the world, it is nothing short of a miracle that they unearth a single gem. However, *Opium* and *Poison* worked for Christian Dior, being words understood in both English and French and doubtless because nobody had ever imagined that they would be suitable names for a perfume. The sweet-sounding, feminine cadence of Givenchy's more traditionally named *Ysatis* was the result of a computer amalgamation of Yseult and Isis. Although in the majority of cases, a name under consideration has already been registered as a trademark, if after five years it has not been used, the registration may expire. More often than not, rights can be obtained by amicable settlement, but the right name can be worth millions of dollars and defensive measures are taken to protect it from imitations – in this way, Dior ring-fenced *Poison* by registering, among others, the names Venom, Vitriol and Serpent.

Another essential factor in a perfume's success is its packaging – the bottle, its box, and even the advertising material. Many bottle designers have followed in the footsteps of Lalique, who was instrumental in Coty's commercial prosperity. The first task of the designer is to understand the personality of the couturier or perfume-maker, immersing themselves in the imaginary world which the perfume must evoke. The second stage involves making the dream real, capturing a mystique in solid materials sometimes resistant to design theory. Numerous models and prototypes have to be made in order to find the exact shade of colored glass, right degree of frosting or perfect shape of stopper required. Glass-makers and molders must then devise a method of industrial-scale production, where financial constraints usually force a compromise on the design. The tension between dream and reality, between creative subtlety and mass production is the designer's lot. Pierre Dinand, creator of the *Opium* bottle, always strives for the best possible symmetry between a fragrance and its bottle. Developing a relationship with the couturier is another essential stage in designing a bottle. This is the case with Serge Mansau, who has found Kenzo a remarkably rich source of inspiration. Far from the rigid and often superficial demands of the marketing team, the dialogue between two artists is the best guarantee of a perfume's success, for the magic of a fine fragrance is a result of this creative dynamic.

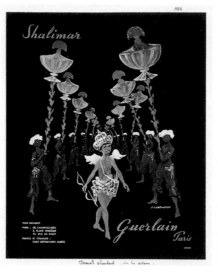
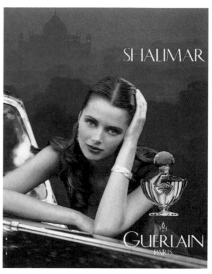

Images of women began to appear in advertisements in the Fifties, and from this time onwards, a specific client group was targeted – the sporty woman, the femme fatale, the executive woman, etc.
The current advertisement for Guerlain's Shalimar *(right) aims for "the boldly sensual and seductive woman," while the "Cupid" (left), designed in 1959 by Charnotet, serves as a reminder that the use of photography in advertising did not become widespread until the Sixties.*

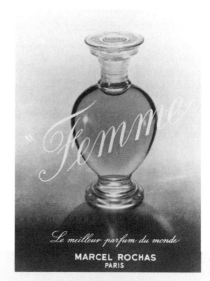

Forty years separate these two advertisements for Femme, *the perfume by Marcel Rochas. It is the quality of the perfume which is emphasized in 1950: "the best perfume in the world." The poster below received the award for the best advertising campaign of 1990.*

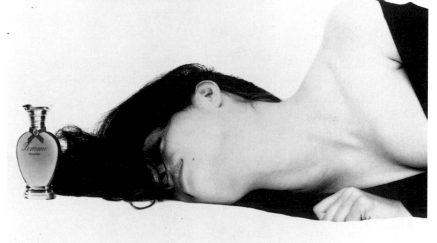

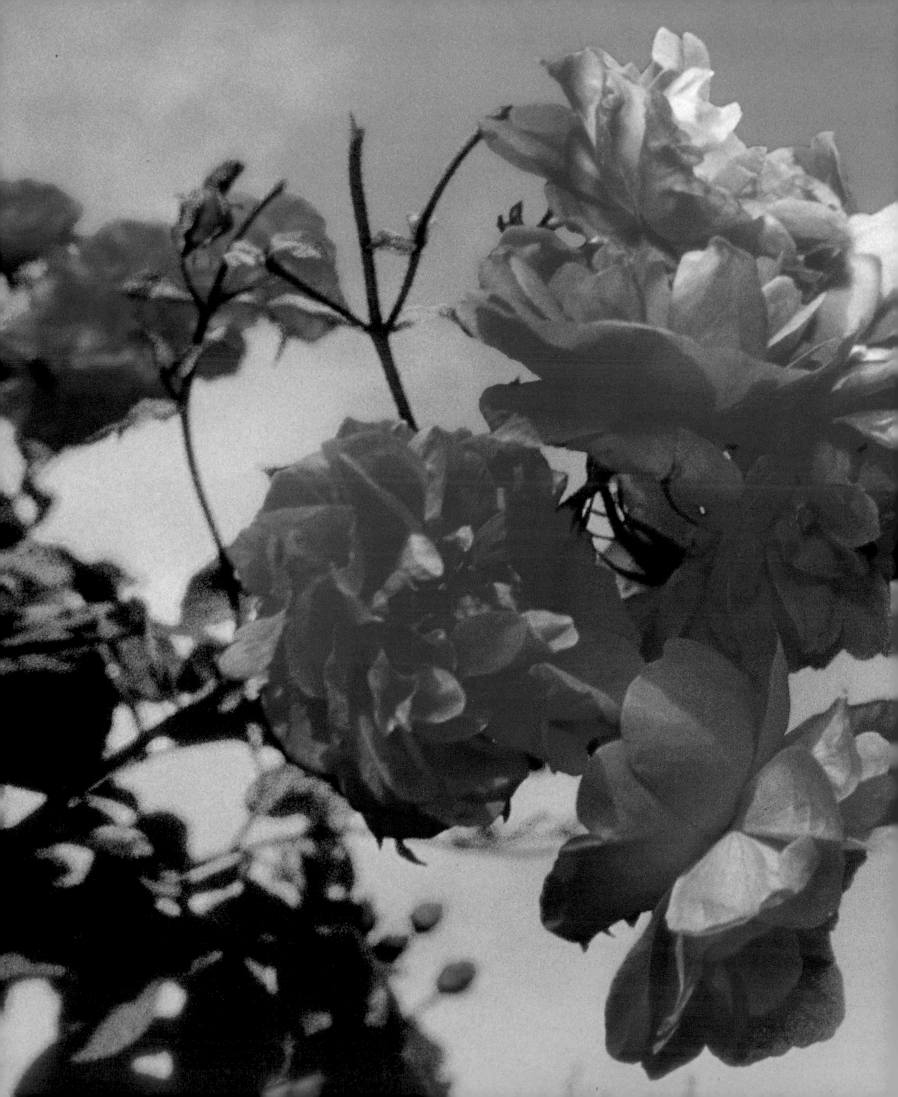

PERFUME CLASSIFICATION

The perfume families, as classified by the technical department of the
Société française des parfumeurs and published by the *Comité français du parfum*.
Use it to discover your favorite perfume's family.

A. THE CITRUS FAMILY

Containing all early eaux de Cologne for men and women, this family features the essential oils obtained by the expression method from the zest of fruits such as lemon, bergamot, orange and grapefruit.

1 ✿ Citrus
2 ✿ Floral Chypre Citrus
3 ✿ Spicy Citrus
4 ✿ Woody Citrus
5 ✿ Aromatic Citrus

B. THE FLORAL FAMILY

This is the largest family, containing perfumes whose principal theme is a flower – rose, jasmine, violet, lilac, lily of the valley, narcissus, tuberose, etc.

1 ✿ Single-fragrance Floral
2 ✿ Lavender
3 ✿ Floral Bouquet
4 ✿ Green Floral
5 ✿ Aldehydic Floral
6 ✿ Woody Floral
7 ✿ Fruity Woody Floral

C. THE FERN FAMILY

The name of this family is purely notional, with no attempt made to reproduce the smell of ferns. These perfumes feature blends usually composed of notes of lavender, wood, oak moss, coumarin, bergamot, etc.

1 ✿ Fern
2 ✿ Sweet Oriental Fern
3 ✿ Flowery Oriental Fern
4 ✿ Spicy Fern
5 ✿ Aromatic Fern

D. THE CHYPRE FAMILY

Named after the perfume created in 1917 by François Coty, which was so successful that it became the principal fragrance in a family of its own, the perfumes featured are mainly based on blends of oak moss, labdanum, patchouli, bergamot, etc.

1 ✿ Chypre
2 ✿ Flowery Chypre
3 ✿ Aldehydic Flowery Chypre
4 ✿ Fruity Chypre
5 ✿ Green Chypre
6 ✿ Aromatic Chypre
7 ✿ Leather Chypre

E. THE WOODY FAMILY

This family comprises perfumes with warm notes, such as sandalwood and patchouli, as well as dry notes like cedar and vetiver, whose base notes are often citrus and lavender blends.

1 ✿ Woody
2 ✿ Citrus Conifer Woody
3 ✿ Aromatic Woody
4 ✿ Spicy Woody
5 ✿ Leather Spicy Woody
6 ✿ Oriental Woody

F. THE ORIENTAL FAMILY

This family groups together compositions with sweet, powdery, vanilla, labdanum and pronounced animal notes. The sub-category of the sweet Orientals is the most representative of the family.

1 ✿ Woody Flowery Oriental
2 ✿ Spicy Flowery Oriental
3 ✿ Sweet Oriental
4 ✿ Citrus Oriental
5 ✿ Flowery Semi-Oriental

G. THE LEATHER FAMILY

Something of a special case in perfume manufacture, this family comprises perfumes featuring dry notes which attempt to reproduce the characteristic smell of leather (smoke, burnt wood, tobacco, etc.) and top notes with floral overtones. As there are so few perfumes of this type, no illustrations are given.

1 ✿ Leather
2 ✿ Flowery Leather
3 ✿ Leather Tobacco

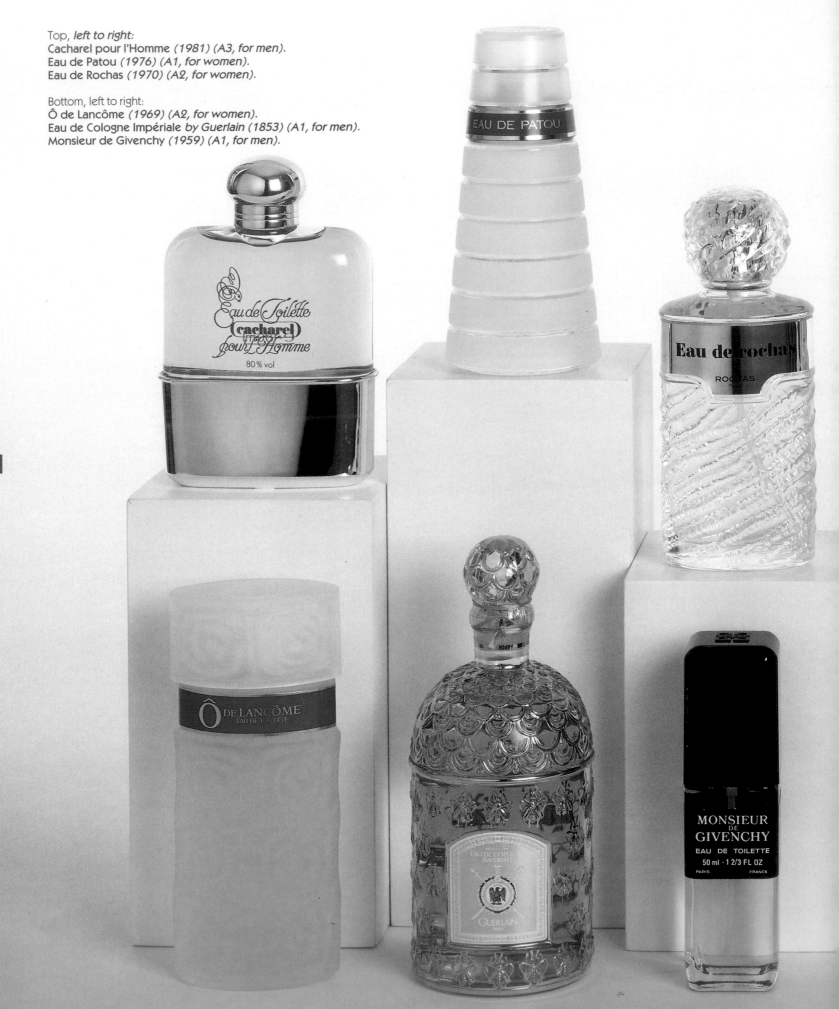

Top, *left to right:*
Cacharel pour l'Homme *(1981) (A3, for men).*
Eau de Patou *(1976) (A1, for women).*
Eau de Rochas *(1970) (A2, for women).*

Bottom, *left to right:*
Ô de Lancôme *(1969) (A2, for women).*
Eau de Cologne Impériale *by Guerlain (1853) (A1, for men).*
Monsieur de Givenchy *(1959) (A1, for men).*

Top, left to right:
Green Water *by Jacques Fath (1947) (A5, for men).*
Eau Sauvage *by Christian Dior (1966) (A2, for men).*
1881 *by Nino Cerruti (1990) (A4, for men).*

Bottom, left to right:
Monsieur Balmain *(1964) (A1, for men).*
Eau Fraîche *by Léonard (1974) (A2, for women).*
Armani *(1984) (A4, for men).*

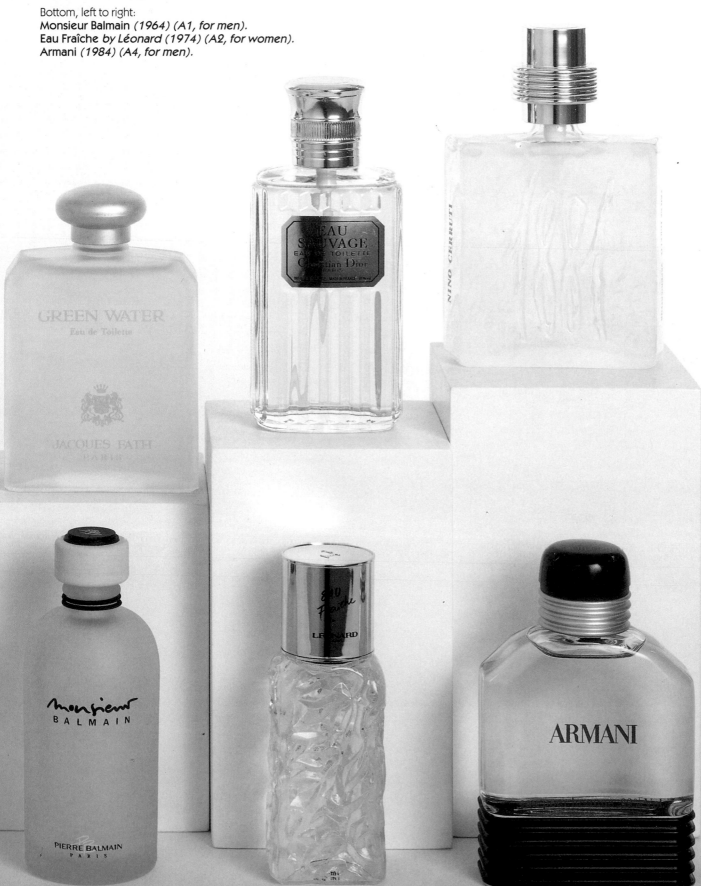

Top, left to right:
L'Air du Temps *by Nina Ricci (1948) (B3, for women).*
Arpège *by Lanvin (1927) (B5 for women).*
Madame Rochas *(1960) (B5, for women).*

Bottom, left to right:
Paris *by Yves Saint Laurent (1983) (B3, for women).*
Le Dix *by Balenciaga (1947) (B3, for women).*
Je Reviens *by Worth (1932) (B3, for women).*

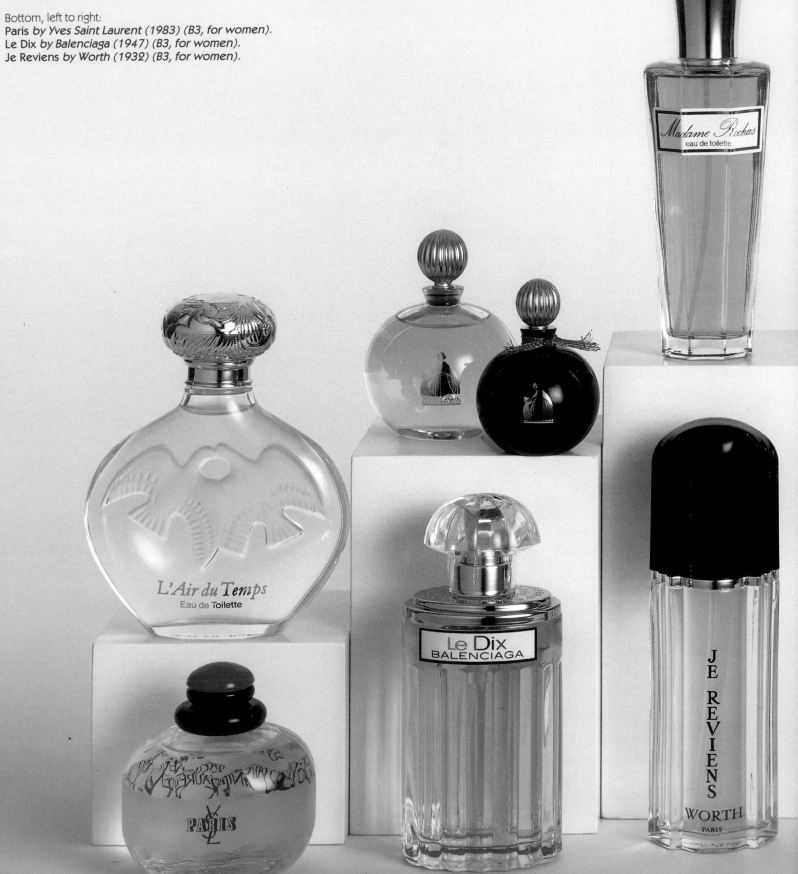

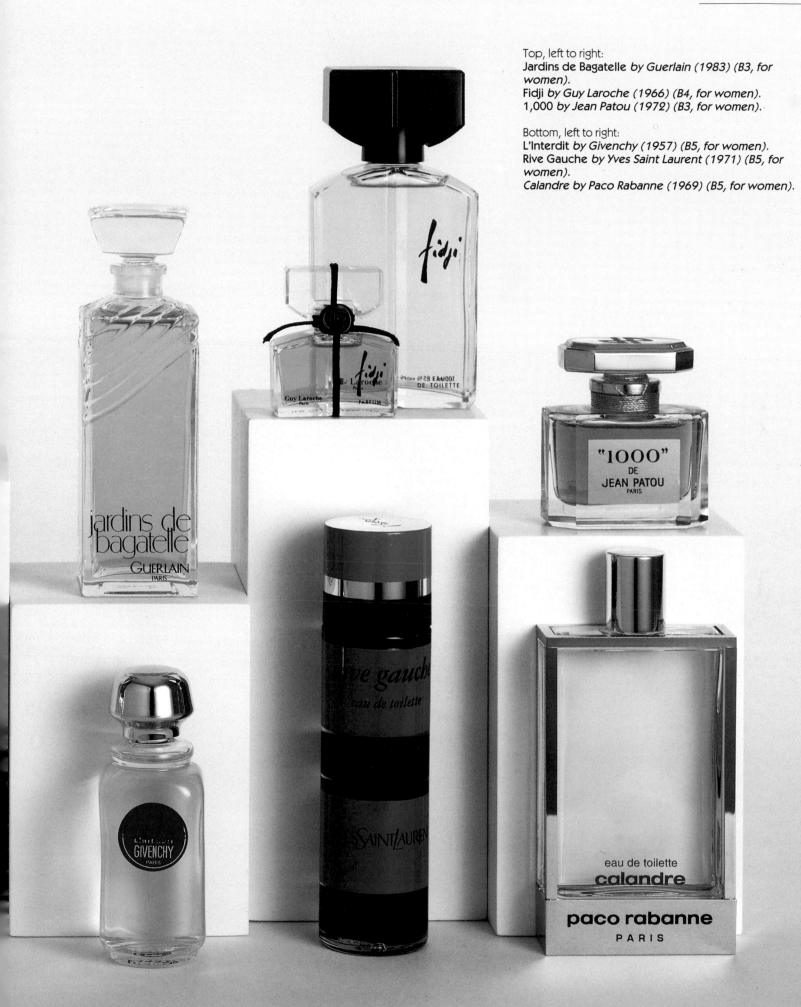

Top, left to right:
Jardins de Bagatelle *by Guerlain (1983) (B3, for women).*
Fidji *by Guy Laroche (1966) (B4, for women).*
1,000 *by Jean Patou (1972) (B3, for women).*

Bottom, left to right:
L'Interdit *by Givenchy (1957) (B5, for women).*
Rive Gauche *by Yves Saint Laurent (1971) (B5, for women).*
Calandre *by Paco Rabanne (1969) (B5, for women).*

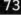

73

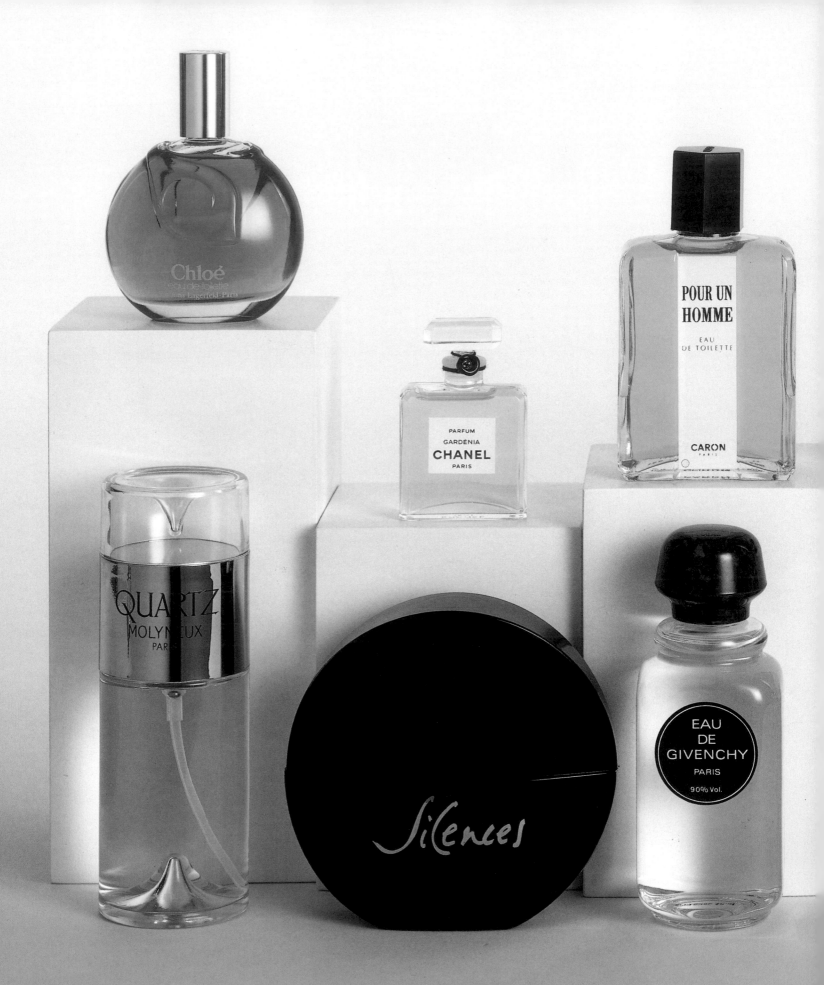

Top, left to right:
Chloé by Karl Lagerfeld (1975) (B1, single fragrance tuberose, for women).
Gardénia by Chanel (1925) (B1, single fragrance gardenia, for women).
Pour un Homme by Caron (1934) (B2, for men).

Bottom, left to right:
Quartz by Molyneux (1977) (B7, for women).
Silences by Jacomo (1978) (B4, for women).
Eau de Givenchy (1980) (B4, for women).

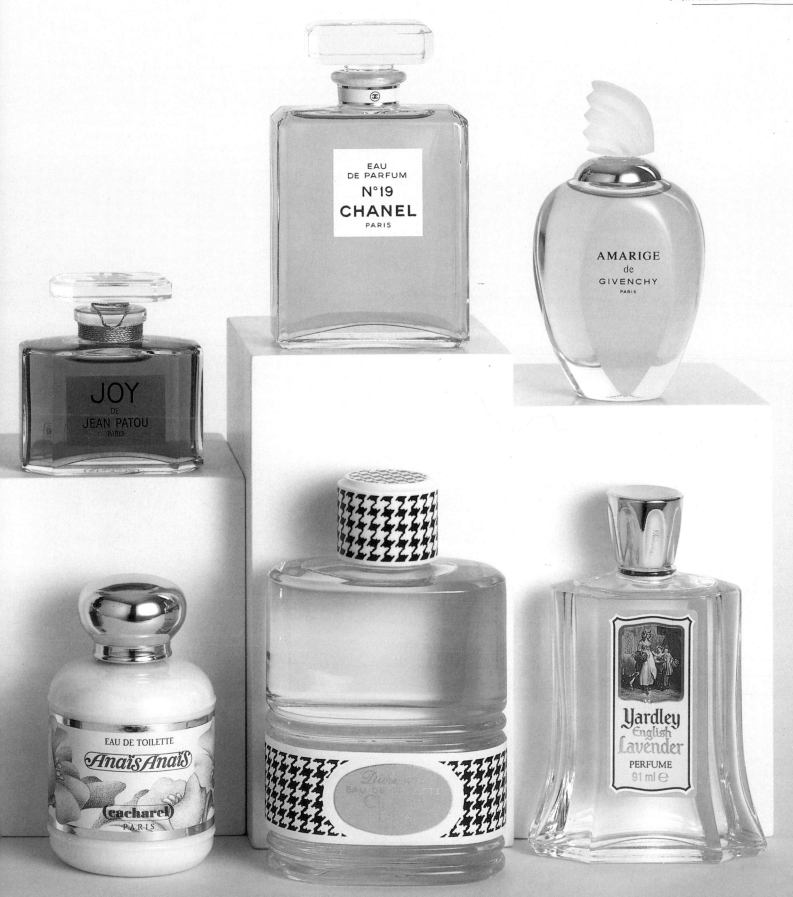

Top, left to right:
Joy by Jean Patou (1930) (B3, for women).
Chanel No.19 (1970) (B4, for women).
Amarige by Givenchy (1991) (B6, for women).

Bottom, left to right:
Anaïs Anaïs by Cacharel (1979) (B3, for women).
Diorissimo by Christian Dior (1956) (B1, single fragrance lily of the valley, for women).
Old English Lavender by Yardley (1913) (B2, for men).

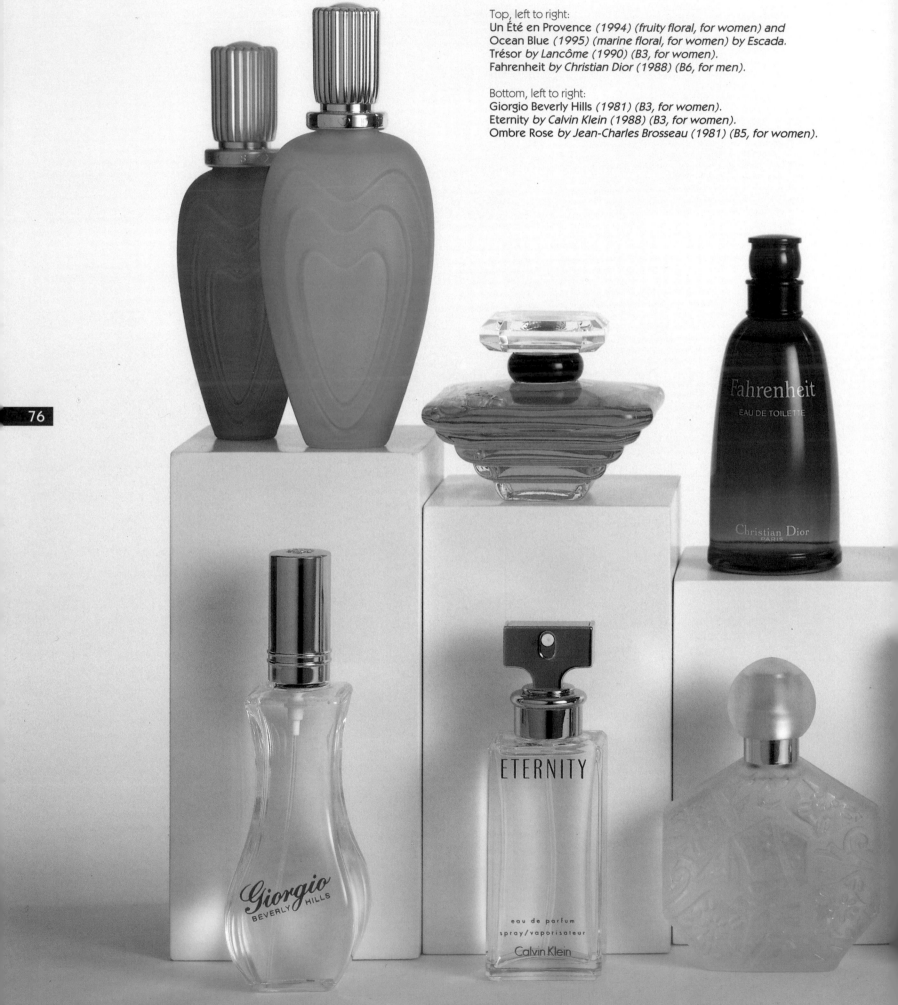

Top, left to right:
Un Été en Provence *(1994) (fruity floral, for women) and*
Ocean Blue *(1995) (marine floral, for women) by Escada.*
Trésor *by Lancôme (1990) (B3, for women).*
Fahrenheit *by Christian Dior (1988) (B6, for men).*

Bottom, left to right:
Giorgio Beverly Hills *(1981) (B3, for women).*
Eternity *by Calvin Klein (1988) (B3, for women).*
Ombre Rose *by Jean-Charles Brosseau (1981) (B5, for women).*

Top, left to right:
Cool Water *by Davidoff (1988) (B7, for men).*
Rose Cardin *(1990) (B7, for women).*
Chanel No.5 *(1921) (B5, for women).*

Bottom, left to right:
Lalique *(1992) (B6, for women).*
Féminité du Bois *by Shisheido (1992) (marine floral, for women).*
Ferre de Ferre *(1990) (B5, for women).*

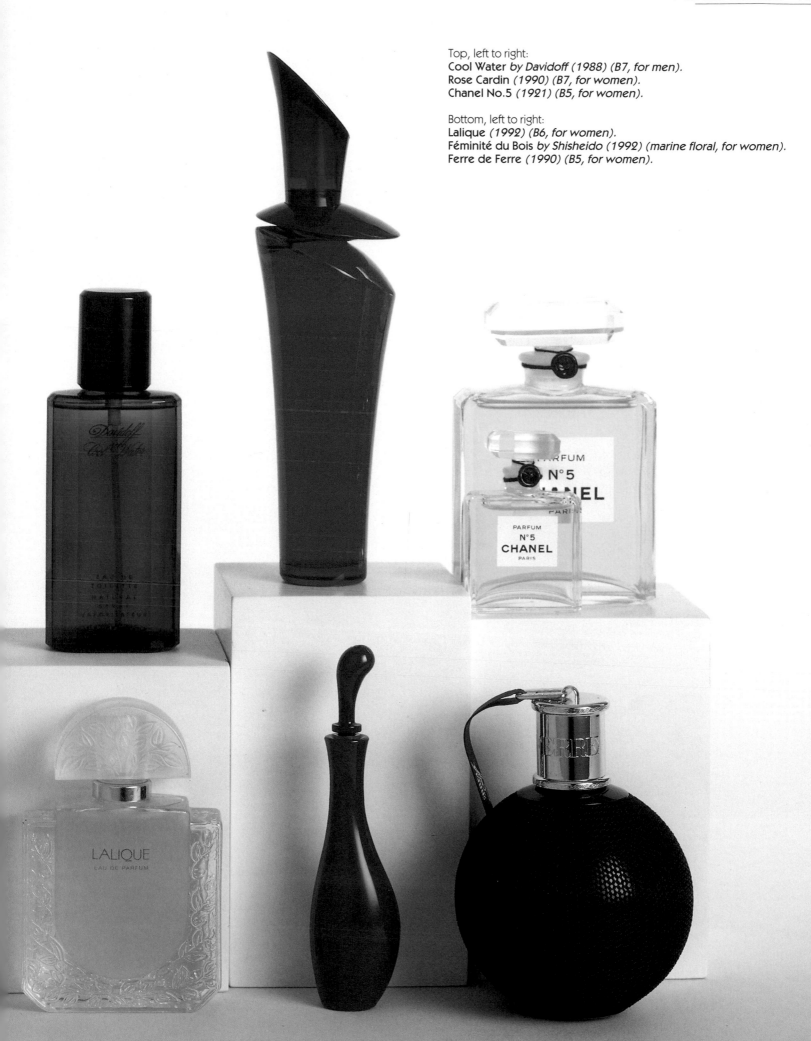

77

Top, left to right:
Monsieur Rochas *(1969) (C4, for men)*.
Canoé *by Dana (1935) (C1, for women)*.
Ho Hang *by Balenciaga (1971) (C4, for men)*.

Bottom, left to right:
Lacoste *(1984) (C5, for men)*.
Drakkar Noir *by Guy Laroche (1982) (C5, for men)*.
Jazz *by Yves Saint Laurent (1988) (C5, for men)*.

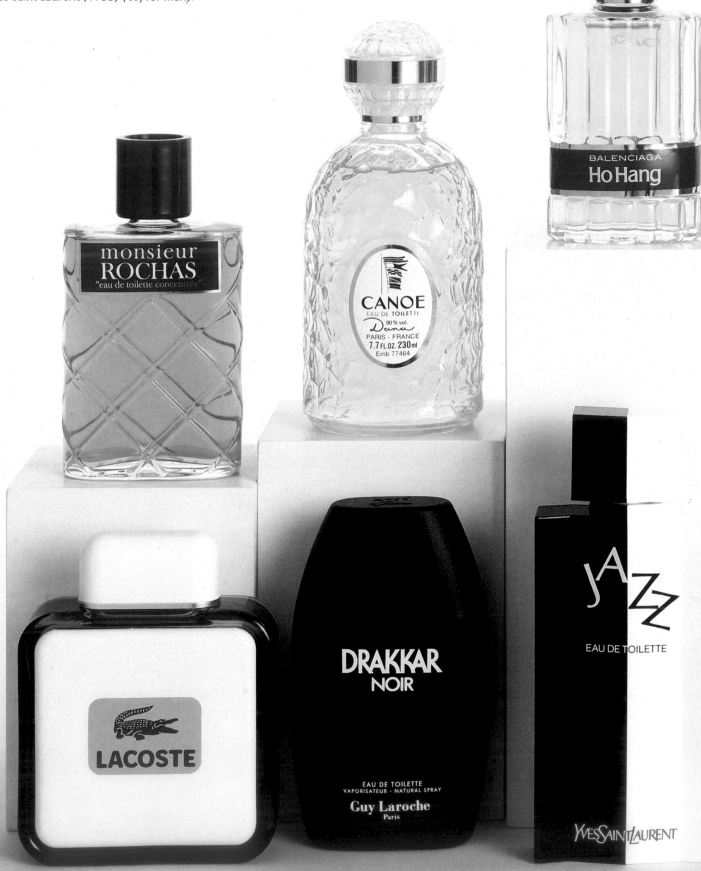

Top, left to right:
Équipage *by Hermès* (1970) (C4, for men).
Boss (1986) (C5, for men).
Rabanne pour Homme (1973) (C5, for men).

Bottom, left to right:
Jicky *by Guerlain* (1889) (C1, for women).
Azzaro pour Homme (1978) (C5, for men).
Captain *by Molyneux* (1975) (C5, for men).

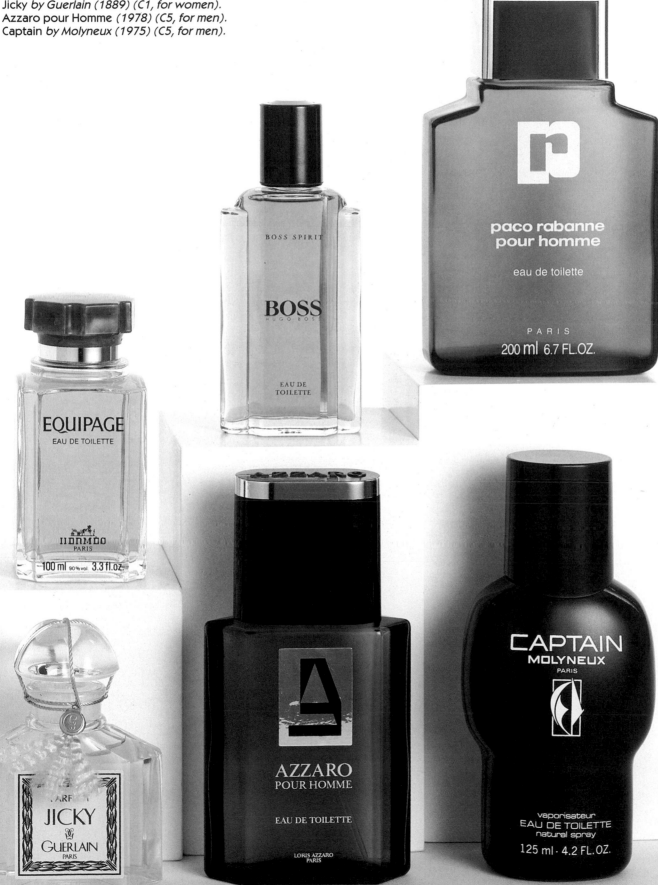

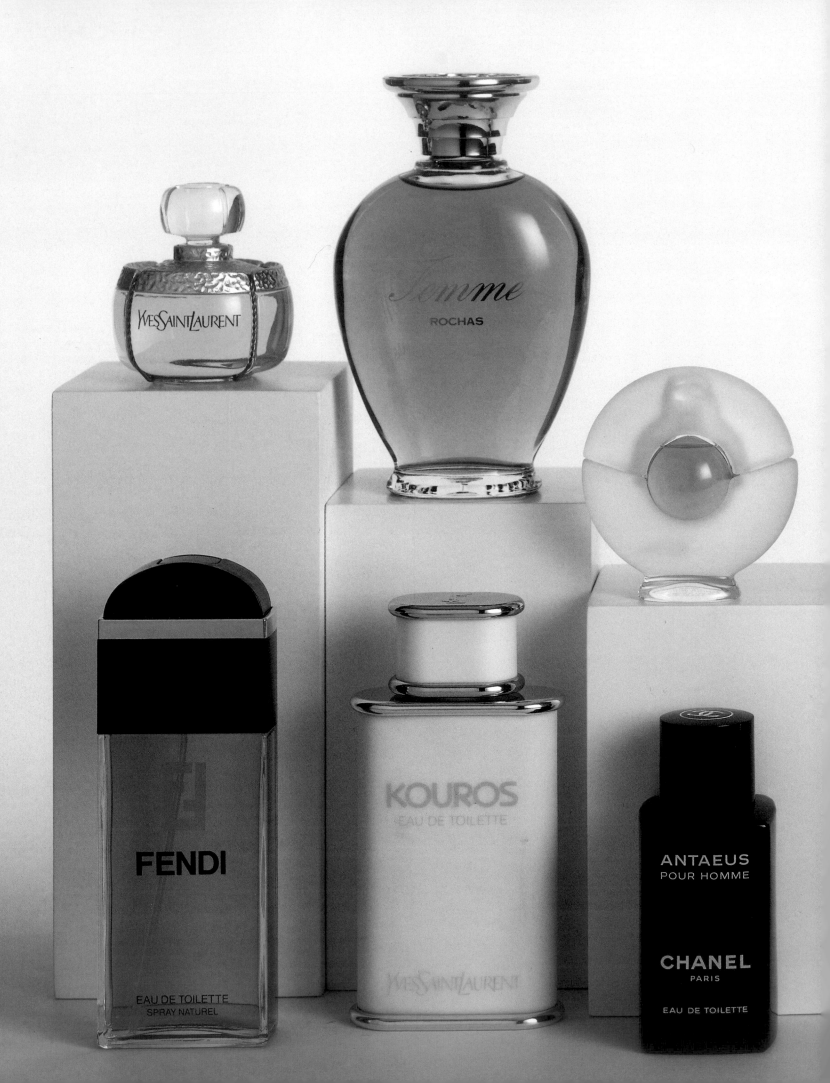

Opposite top, left to right:
Yves Saint Laurent *(1993) (D4, for women).*
Femme *by Rochas (1944) (D4, for women).*
Paloma Picasso *(1985) (D3, for women).*
Opposite bottom, left to right:
Fendi *(1987) (D3, for women).*
Kouros *by Yves Saint Laurent (1981) (D6, for men).*
Antaeus pour Homme *by Chanel (1981) (D7, for men).*

Top, left to right:
Mitsouko *by Guerlain (1919) (D4, for women).*
Coriandre *by Jean Couturier (1973) (D3, for women).*
Diva *by Emmanuel Ungaro (1983) (D3, for women).*
Bottom, left to right:
Empreinte *by Courrèges (1971) (D7, for women).*
Miss Dior *(1947) (D5, for women).*
Ma Griffe *by Carven (1946) (D3, for women).*

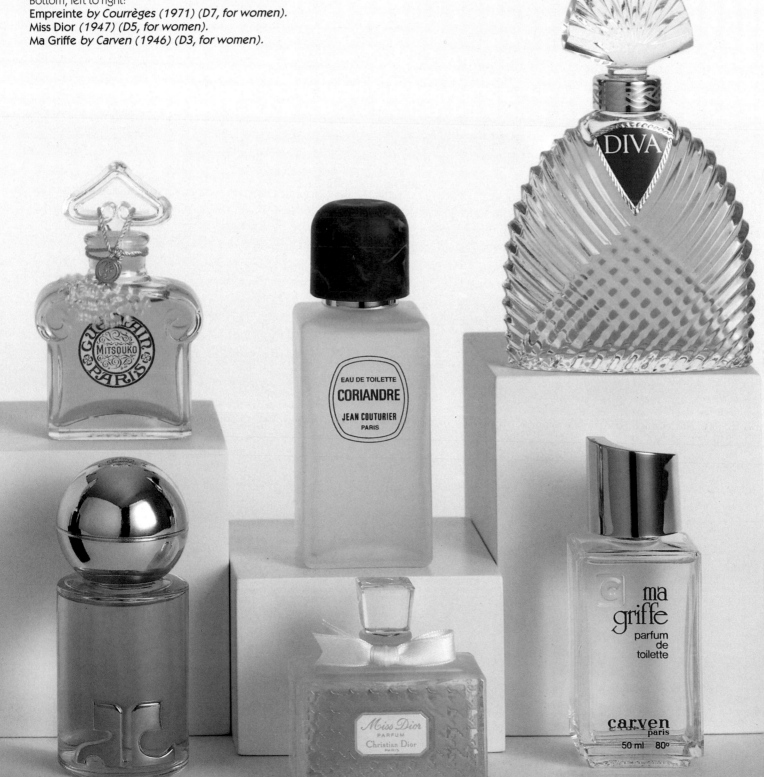

Top, left to right:
Minotaure *by Paloma Picasso (1992) (E6, for men).*
Vetiver *by Guerlain (1959) (E4, for men).*
Ricci Club *(1989) (E4, for men).*

Bottom, left to right:
Jacomo de Jacomo *(1980) (E4, for men).*
Vetiver *by Carven (1957) (E1, for men).*
Gentleman *by Givenchy (1974) (E6, for men).*

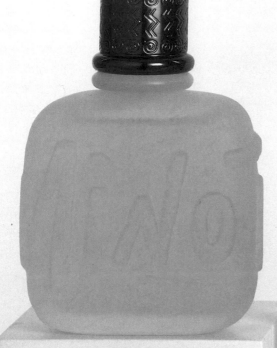

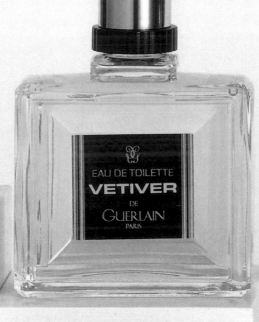

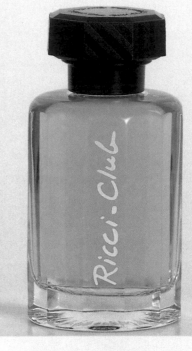

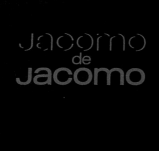

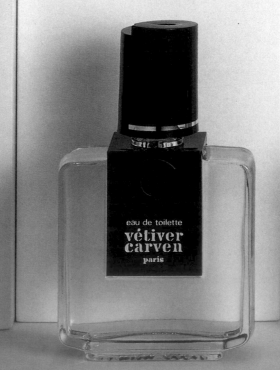

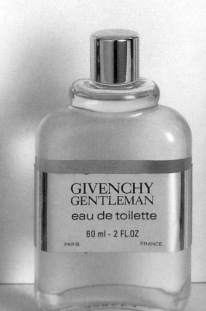

Top, left to right:
Safari for Men by Ralph Lauren (1992) (E3).
Kenzo pour Homme (1991) (marine woody, for men).
Égoïste by Chanel (1990) (E4, for men).

Bottom, left to right:
Versace l'Homme (1984) (E3, for men).
One Man Show by Jacques Bogart (1980) (E3, for men).
Xeryus by Givenchy (1986) (E3, for men).

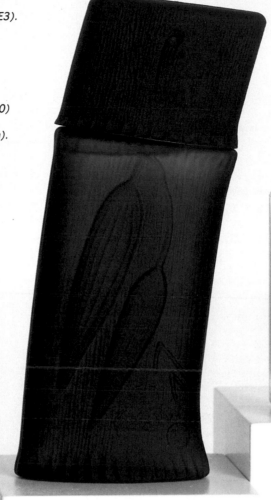

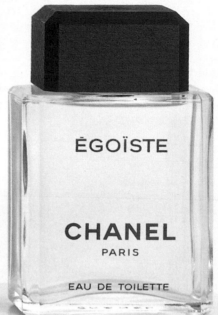

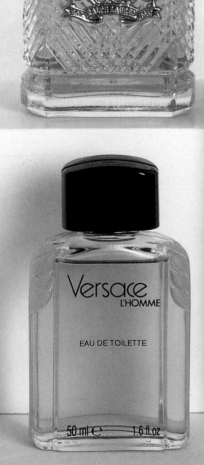

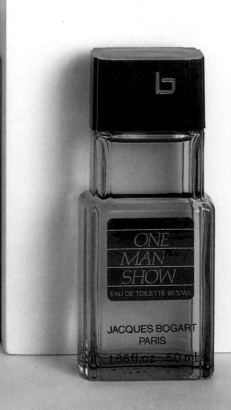

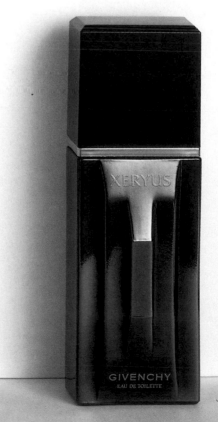

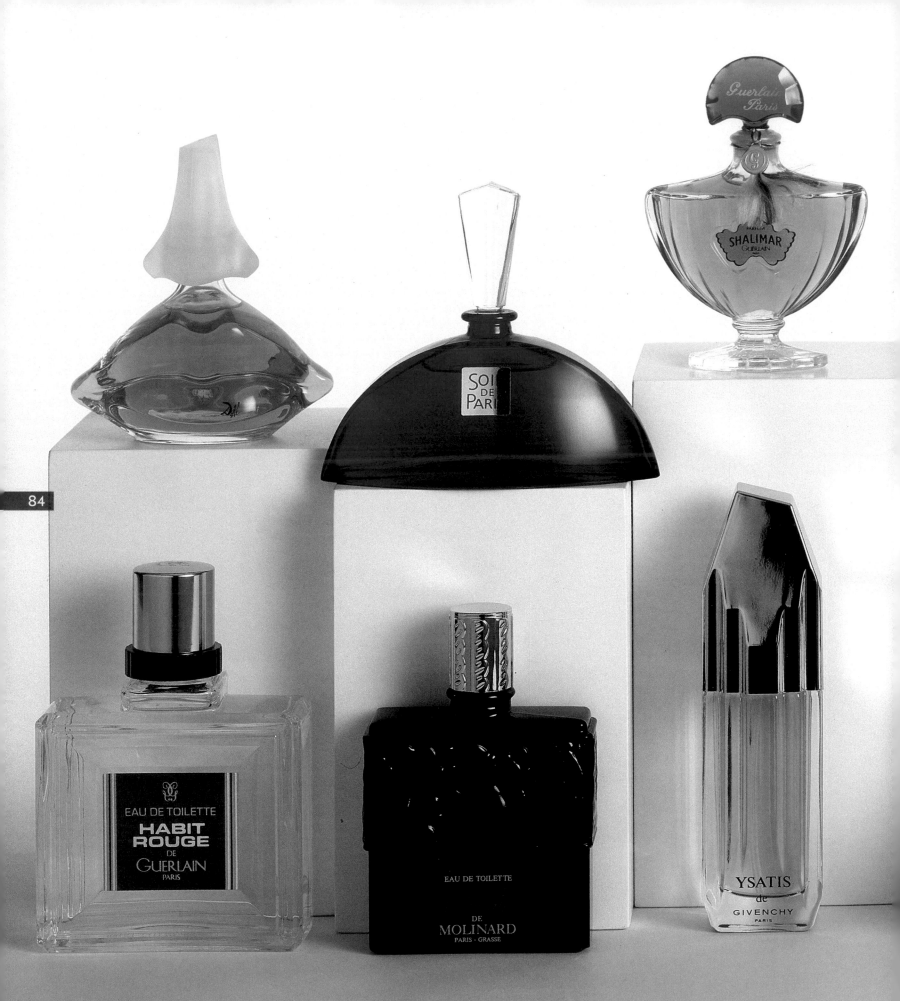

Top, left to right:
Dali by Salvador Dali (1984) (F1, for women).
Soir de Paris by Bourjois (1928) (F2, for women).
Shalimar by Guerlain (1925) (F3, for women).

Bottom, left to right:
Habit Rouge by Guerlain (1965) (F4, for men).
Habanita by Molinard (1924) (F1, for women).
Ysatis by Givenchy (1984) (F1, for women).

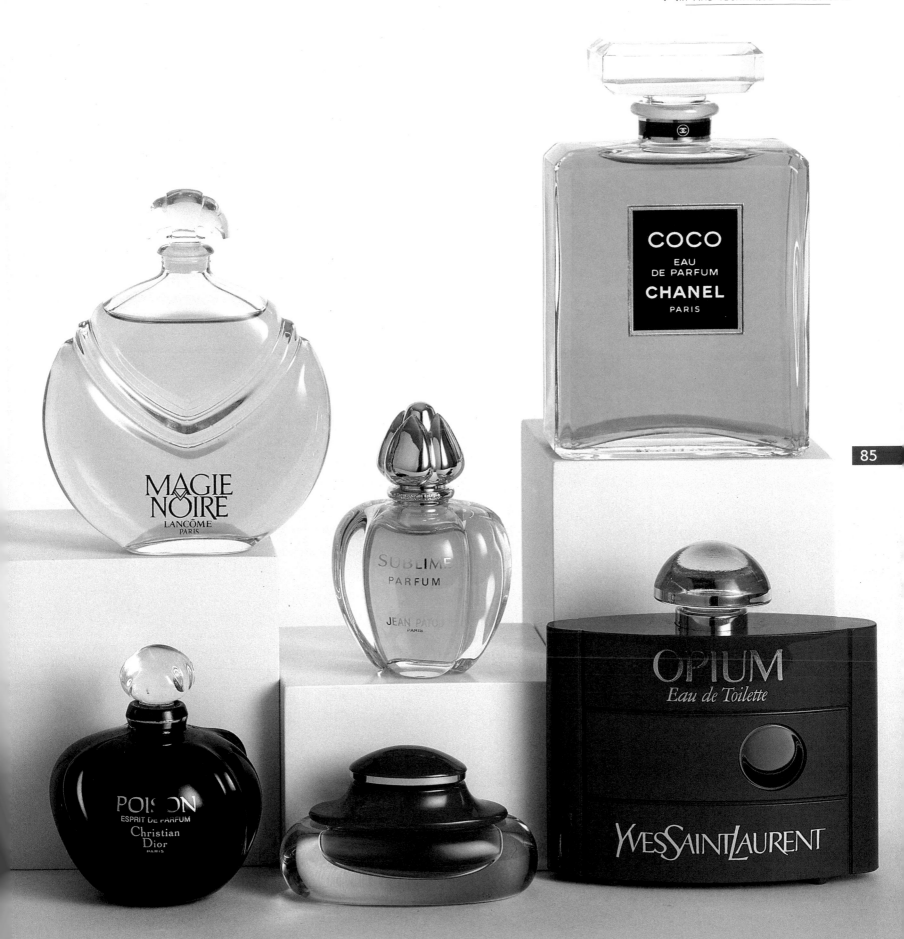

Top, left to right:
Magie Noire by Lancôme (1978) (F1, for women).
Sublime by Jean Patou (1992) (F5, for women).
Coco by Chanel (1984) (F5, for women).

Bottom, left to right:
Poison by Christian Dior (1985) (F2, for women).
Obsession by Calvin Klein (1985) (F1, for women).
Opium by Yves Saint Laurent (1977) (F5, for women).

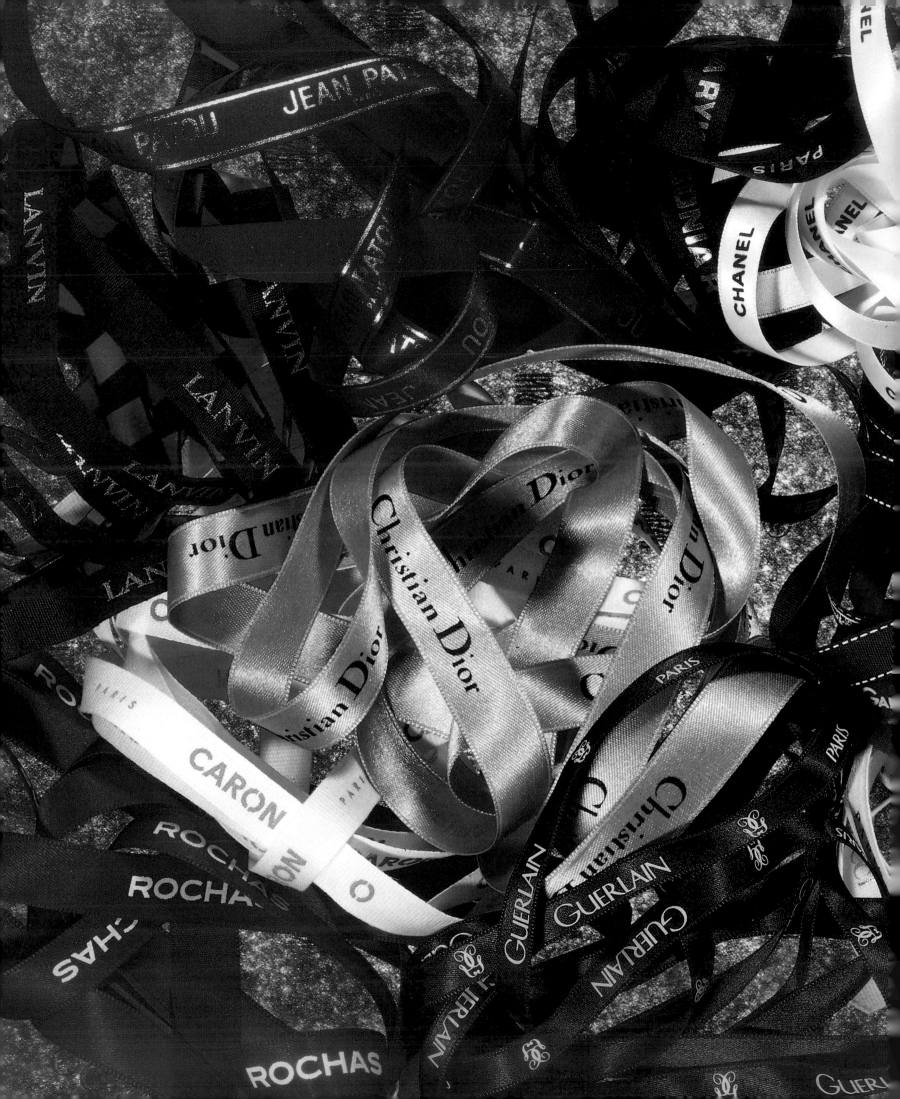

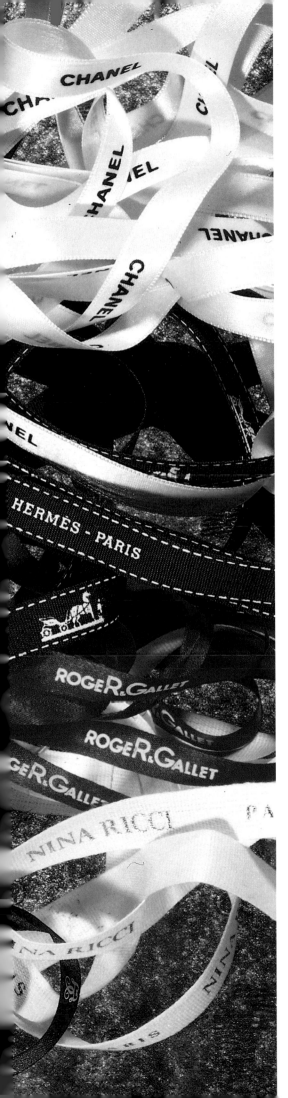

THE GREAT NAMES OF PERFUMERY

Fine perfumes have long been associated with the name of a famous couturier, jeweler or leather goods maker – today, Guerlain and Lancôme are among the few remaining sole manufacturers of perfume. The fusion of perfume-maker with couturier began in the early years of this century, with Paul Poiret being the first to market his own perfume as a sophisticated extension of his clothing designs. Perhaps because he had christened the new business *Les Parfums de Rosine*, after one of his daughters, and his name did not appear on the bottles, his idea failed somewhat to realize its financial potential. In 1921, Coco Chanel followed in his footsteps with her world renowned *No.5*, this time understanding the benefits of putting her name to her fragrances. Her decision was validated by the long list of couturiers – Worth, Jeanne Lanvin, Jean Patou, Molyneux, Lucien Lelong, Elsa Schiaparelli, Robert Piguet, Carven, Marcel Rochas and Pierre Balmain – who would follow the same path.

When Christian Dior established his couture business in 1947, he immediately grasped the importance of accompanying the launch with a perfume *(Miss Dior)*. The same year saw the appearance of the first perfumes from Nina Ricci *(Cœur Joie)* and Balenciaga *(Le Dix)*. From the Fifties onwards, new names were added to the illustrious list – Hubert de Givenchy, Pierre Cardin, Courrèges, Yves Saint Laurent, Louis Féraud, Guy Laroche, Paco Rabanne and the leather goods maker Hermès. More recently, designers such as Kenzo, Claude Montana, Jean-Paul Gaultier, Thierry Mugler and, in a different style, Christian Lacroix have proved no exception to the rule. The imagination and daring which characterizes their collections is also frequently found in their perfumes.

As far back as the Thirties, this constant quest for innovation led Colette to write, "Thanks to the couturier, perfume can become something more than a mere sound in an elegant orchestral arrangement: it can and must represent the melody, the clear and direct expression of the trends and tastes of our time." Contemporary couturiers would do well to remember these words, but must also bear in mind that the quality of a perfume is measured by its longevity, whereas fashion is dictated by transience and renewal.

Couturiers, jewelers and leather goods makers: all responsible for the most famous perfumes of the twentieth century.

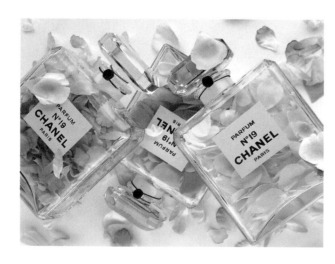

Chanel is one of the only perfume manufacturers that makes its own essences and concretes. This practice has led this great company to re-invest in growing plants for its exclusive use, as in the case of the famous May roses from Grasse used in the composition of many Chanel perfumes.

No.19 – created in 1970 by Henri Robert, the perfume derives its name from Coco Chanel's birthday.

CHANEL
THE STYLISTIC REVOLUTION

It was undoubtedly memories of her childhood which, towards the end of her life, prompted Gabrielle Chanel to say, "If you are born without wings, don't stop any from growing." Little is known about the early years of the "Grande Mademoiselle," apart from the fact that her mother died when she was twelve and that she was left by her father in the care of an orphanage in central France. As a teenager she quickly developed a tough character with a strong independent streak and, once she had left school, she began work as a shop assistant at a hosiers in Moulins. In her spare time, she sang at *La Rotonde*, a concert hall popular with officers from the regiment stationed nearby. Her repertoire comprised two songs, *Ko Ko Ri Ko* and *Qui qu'a vu Coco?*, and her admirers were quick to give her a nickname derived from the element common to both – the legend of Coco was born.

In 1910, Chanel established her workshop in rue Cambon in Paris – the sign outside read "Chanel, Milliner." Some years earlier, she had been plucked from her provincial life by Étienne Balsan, a wealthy young man who offered her a life of luxury and leisure. However, Coco soon tired of the easy life and when Boy Capel, who was Étienne's best friend and later became her lover, agreed to help her finance a hat shop in Paris, she did not hesitate for a moment.

Having established her reputation as a hat-maker, she soon introduced her own line of clothing, initially creating a style which did not then exist for women – sportswear. She paraded herself on the beach, wearing a woollen fisherman's smock and flowing skirt at a time when knitwear was considered unfashionable. In 1913, she opened her first boutique in Deauville, soon frequented by a faithful clientele, and the simple, practical and elegant Chanel style emerged. With the outbreak of war in 1914, the clothes worn by these women had to adapt to new circumstances and Chanel's first loose-cut suit, worn without a corset, was the ideal solution. Two years later, she introduced jersey into the collection, designing a coat which had no belt or decoration and disguised the bust and hips under severe, almost masculine lines. She also created the "charming chemise dress" so rapturously received by *Harper's Bazaar*. After Paul Poiret, the great turn of the century couturier, had lifted hemlines to reveal the feet, she went further and showed the ankle. The rest is history. Women flocked to Chanel boutiques, soon regarded as the epitome of style. One evening, she arrived at the Opéra in Paris with her hair cut short, and legend has it that thirty-five thousand salons opened in France as a result. The moment that she wore round-toed shoes, women threw out their terrible pointed, three-strap shoes. She wore pearls over her sweater and every woman copied her. She would try anything, even daring to expose her face to the sun at a time when a tanned complexion was regarded as vulgar. This innovative spirit led her to instigate many fashions: the dropped waist, trousers for women, beach pyjamas, the famous little black dress which Americans called "Chanel's Model-T Ford," the pleated skirt, the raincoat, the gold-buttoned blazer, suits in Scottish tweed, costume jewelery, long strings of pearls, shoulder bags, quilted handbags with gold-chained straps, black-toed beige court shoes, hair bows, and not to forget the famous Chanel suit, copied the world over, which has become a household name.

Perfume is, of course, the one important element missing from this list which could not have eluded Chanel's creative genius. Coco was fond of quoting her friend Paul Valéry, who said, "A woman without perfume has no future." She wanted to banish the taste for powdery, insipid creations smelling of violets. Her perfume would be unique, unlike any other. For this she enlisted the help of Ernest Beaux, the greatest perfume-blender of the day, whose liberal use of aldehydes, powerful synthetic substances usually administered in only very small quantities, proved exceptionally successful. Blended with natural essences, they gave *No.5* that indefinable quality which immediately established Chanel's first perfume as the precursor to all the great aldehydic floral fragrances. Its reputation spread rapidly beyond France and when Paris was liberated, G.I.s who wanted to take a bottle of *No.5* back to the United States could be seen queuing round the block from her perfume shop. When asked by journalists what she wore in bed, Marilyn Monroe whispered, "A few drops of *No.5*." Later immortalized by the faces of Catherine Deneuve and Carole Bouquet, *No.5* has become one of the legendary symbols of our age, and was followed by *No.22*, then *Cuir de Russie, Gardenia* and *Bois des Îles*. All these compositions were re-designed in 1983 by Jacques Polge, the house "nose." Meanwhile, *Cristalle, No.19*, named after Chanel's birthday, *Pour Monsieur* and *Antaeus* appeared. In 1984, Polge made a dazzling addition to the range with *Coco,* whose dominant spicy notes have left a lasting impression on the perfume industry. In 1990, Chanel launched *Égoïste,* a fragrance for men with the intense notes of Mysore sandalwood (from Karnataka, India), whose originality was matched by Goude's advertising campaign. Six years later, the most recent Chanel creation appeared, *Allure.* When war broke out, Chanel closed her couture shop and was not to re-open it until fifteen years later, by which time Dior's "New Look" had revolutionized fashion. Chanel quickly re-established a success which the company has enjoyed ever since. It was perhaps her friend, the writer Paul Morand, who identified the secret of this success when he described her as having "the kind of robust appetite for revenge which triggers revolutions."

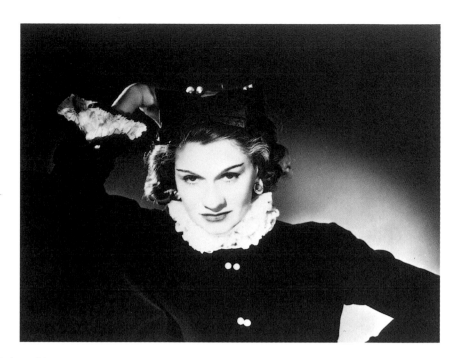

Gabrielle Chanel photographed by Hoyningen Huene in 1935. She single-handedly revolutionized the world of women's fashion and the list of the famous "Mademoiselle's" daring innovations is endless – the use of jersey, the chemise dress, shorter skirts, loosely-fitted suits worn without a corset, short hair, trousers, sportswear and so on.

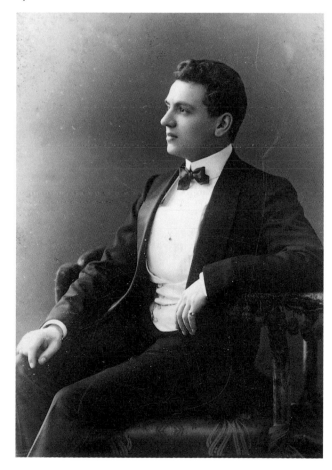

Ernest Beaux, whose partnership with Coco Chanel produced one of the most innovative fragrances in the history of perfumery. He aimed to unite chemistry and nature, creating a work of art through science. He succeeded in 1921 with No.5. A true innovation is immune to the passage of time and so becomes a classic.

Top:
No.5, created in 1921 by the perfume-blender
Ernest Beaux.

Bottom:
No.22, created in 1922, also by Ernest Beaux.
No.5 (as sold).

Top:
Coco, created in 1984 by Chanel's in-house perfume-blender Jacques Polge.
No.19, created in 1970 by Henri Robert.

Bottom:
Gardénia (1925), Bois des Îles (1926) and Cuir de Russie (1924).
All three compositions, created by Ernest Beaux, were re-designed in 1983 by Jacques Polge. They are sold exclusively in Chanel boutiques.

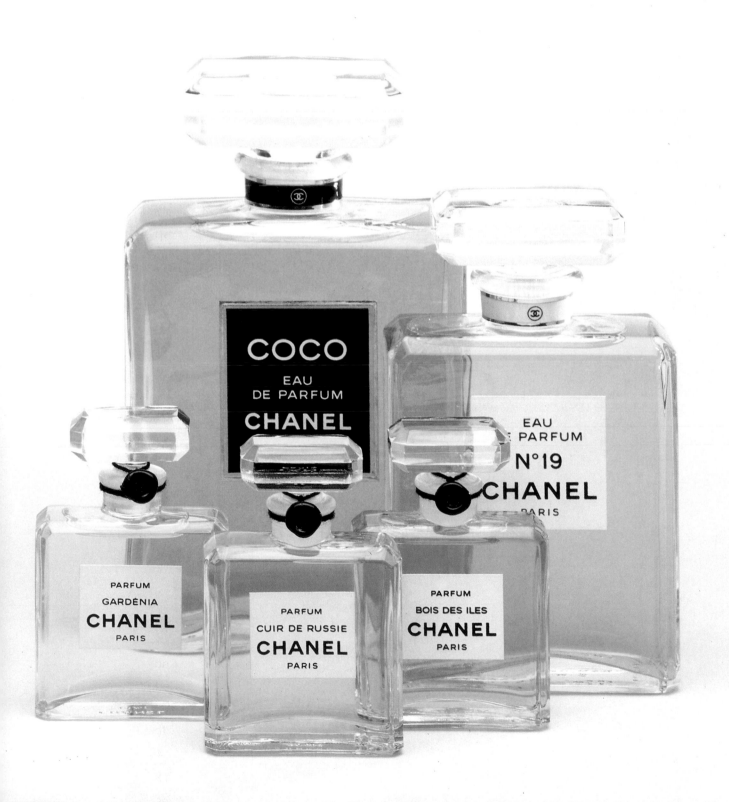

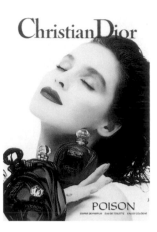

CHRISTIAN DIOR

THE BIRTH OF THE NEW LOOK

"I want to establish a small, discreet couture house for a hand-picked selection of truly elegant women…" It was with these words that the forty-one year old Christian Dior persuaded the great textile magnate Marcel Boussac to lend him the money for his couture business. On February 12, 1947, as Paris shivered in sub-zero temperatures, the designer presented his first collection in a salon on the Avenue Montaigne. An invited audience was shown ninety designs, defined by two title themes: "Huit" ("Eight"), featuring tiny waists and curvaceous hips; and "Corolles," featuring plunging necklines and calf-length skirts. The models paraded endless yards of material as they came down the catwalk.

As France entered the post-war boom and Fifties modernism appeared on the horizon, Dior resurrected fashion in glamorous style. The revolution that he instigated was based on tradition – while shapes remained classic, he give them innovative twists and touches of eccentricity. His fame quickly spread beyond Paris and he was featured on the cover of *Time* magazine. A huge press campaign was organized, culminating in the now legendary words of Carmel Snow, editor-in-chief of *Harper's Bazaar*: "It's a revolution, dear Christian, your dresses have such a new look…"

With the "New Look," a legend was born, and with it the greatest fashion empire in the world. At over forty years of age, Dior was no longer a novice in business. Born to rich industrialists in Granville, Normandy, in 1905, he studied economics in order to please his family. Meanwhile, he nurtured a certain innate instinct for creativity by mixing with Parisian artists like the painter Christian Bérard, the musician Henri Sauguet and the writer Pierre Gaxotte, all three of whom remained among his closest friends. In 1928, he opened a gallery, exhibiting the work of influential artists like Picasso and Fernand Léger, but the stock market collapse of 1929 brought financial ruin to his family and Dior was forced to close shop. He was then taught the techniques of fashion design by a friend and was soon selling his sketches to newspapers and a few major couturiers. He was mobilized in 1939, rejoining his family after the war in the south of France, where he became a farmer for a while. It was here that he was discovered by Lucien Lelong, one of the most famous couturiers of the time, and brought back to Paris as his head designer.

Dior began to enjoy a pleasant, soon to be affluent, existence, dividing his time between work, friends and an enviable lifestyle incorporating good food, fine art and weekends in the country. Now guaranteed a comfortable and trouble-free life, he became a regular feature of the international social scene, celebrated by some and criticized by others in

Maurice Roger, managing director of Christian Dior Perfumes since 1982 and the imagination behind Poison, Fahrenheit and Tendre Poison. Since 1987, Christian Dior Perfumes has been part of the LVMH (Louis Vuitton – Moët Hennessy) group, a symbol of quality and prestige.

the way that all great visionaries are. In America, Nieman Marcus awarded the young couturier fashion's equivalent of an Oscar. Known as "the man who hides women's legs...," with hemlines only a few inches from the ground, he finally impressed the most conservative of his peers, who soon began to imitate him. Dior became a symbol of luxury and elegance regained, making Paris once again the home of the beautiful dress.

Soon after his Paris show, he went to New York to open his own shop on Fifth Avenue. In less than five years, his business acumen had enabled him to create a real empire, whose structure would be borrowed and copied by many other great fashion houses.

This success could not have been complete without the setting up, in 1947, of Christian Dior Perfumes, whose managing director, Serge Heftler Louiche, was a childhood friend of the couturier. Their first creation highlighted the bonds of friendship between the two men. "Serge's ideas were similar to my own," Dior declared. "We worked together for four years, experimenting like alchemists in search of the philosopher's stone." The result was called simply *Miss Dior*, a marvellous Chypre fragrance in perfect harmony with the New Look. "I created this perfume to shroud each woman with desire, to see the essence of my clothes emerge from its bottle," the couturier explained. In the year that it was launched, the Baccarat crystal bottle for *Miss Dior* appeared in a limited edition of just two hundred.

Dior believed that a perfume should express the spirit of the age, reflecting the aspirations and moods of its time while remaining apart from changes in fashion. *Diorama* (1949), *Eau Fraîche* (1953), *Diorissimo* (1956) and *Diorling* (1963) lived up to this ideal. In 1966, Dior again aroused excitement with his first fragrance for men, *Eau Sauvage*, created by Edmond Roudnitska and which has since become a classic. This was followed by *Diorella* (1972), *Dioressence* (1979), *Jules* (1980) and *Eau Sauvage Extrême* (1984). Dior struck a further creative coup in 1985, with the launch of *Poison*. Regarded as a "terrorist" fragrance by some and an unforgettable perfume by others, *Poison* enjoyed huge success and was to remain one of the most emblematic perfumes of the Eighties. Finally, recent years have seen the creation of *Fahrenheit* (1988), for men, and for women, *Dune* (1991), with its hints of the sea, and *Tendre Poison* (1994), a lighter fragrance than its "elder sister."

Dior died in 1957, after only ten years of international fame as a legend in haute couture. The shock waves that he created in the French fashion and luxury industries will continue to be felt for generations to come.

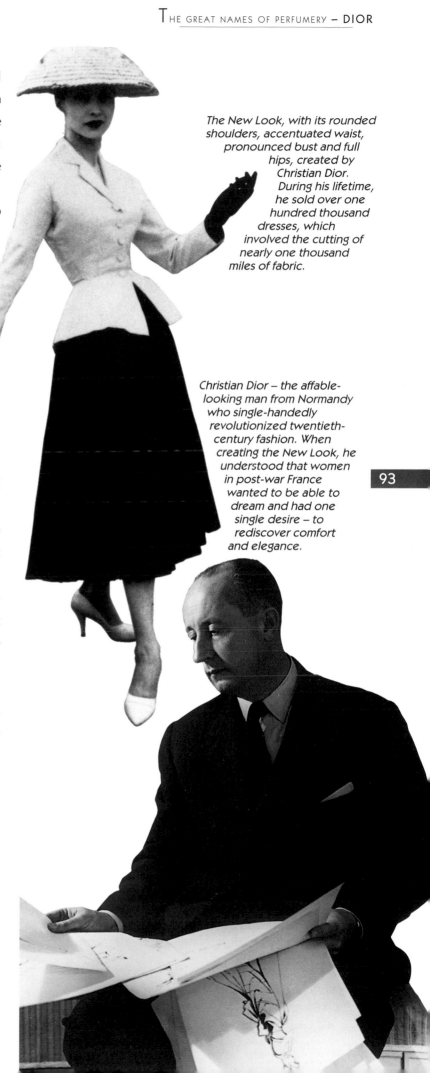

The New Look, with its rounded shoulders, accentuated waist, pronounced bust and full hips, created by Christian Dior. During his lifetime, he sold over one hundred thousand dresses, which involved the cutting of nearly one thousand miles of fabric.

Christian Dior – the affable-looking man from Normandy who single-handedly revolutionized twentieth-century fashion. When creating the New Look, he understood that women in post-war France wanted to be able to dream and had one single desire – to rediscover comfort and elegance.

93

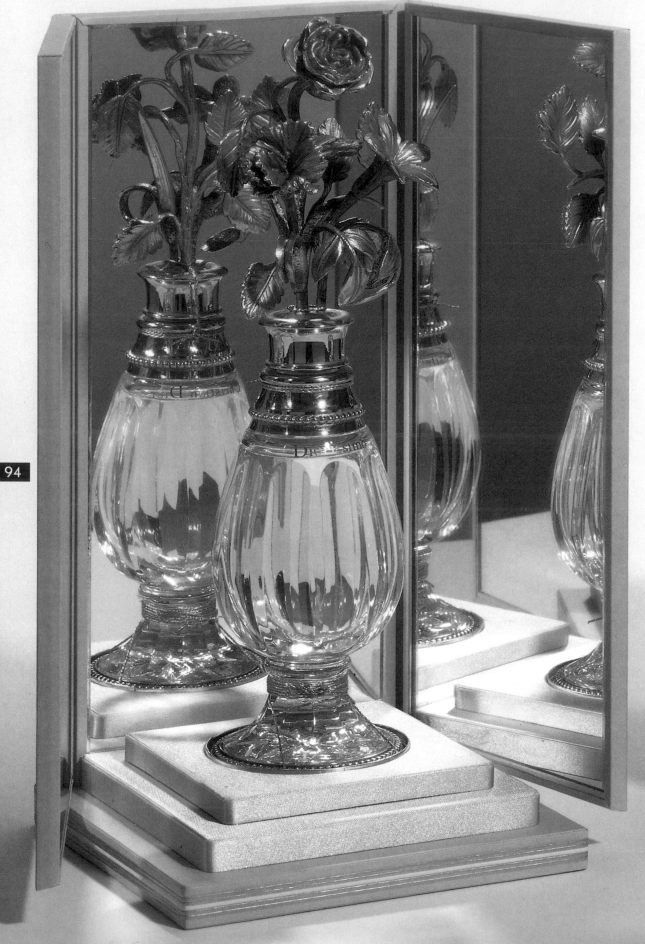

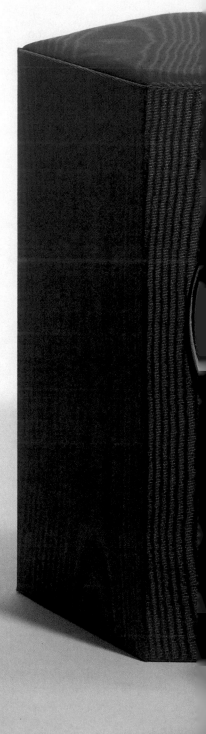

Diorissimo – *Limited edition of the perfume launched in 1956. Baccarat crystal bottle in the shape of an upturned amphora, stopper decorated with a superb gilded bronze bouquet of flowers. The bronze-work, with outstandingly rare quality and detail, was designed and produced by Chrystian Charles.*

Poison – *Limited edition of the perfume launched in 1985. One of the most spectacular successes in the history of perfumery. It has won many awards, including "Best Perfume of 1985" and the New York Fragrance Foundation Oscar.*

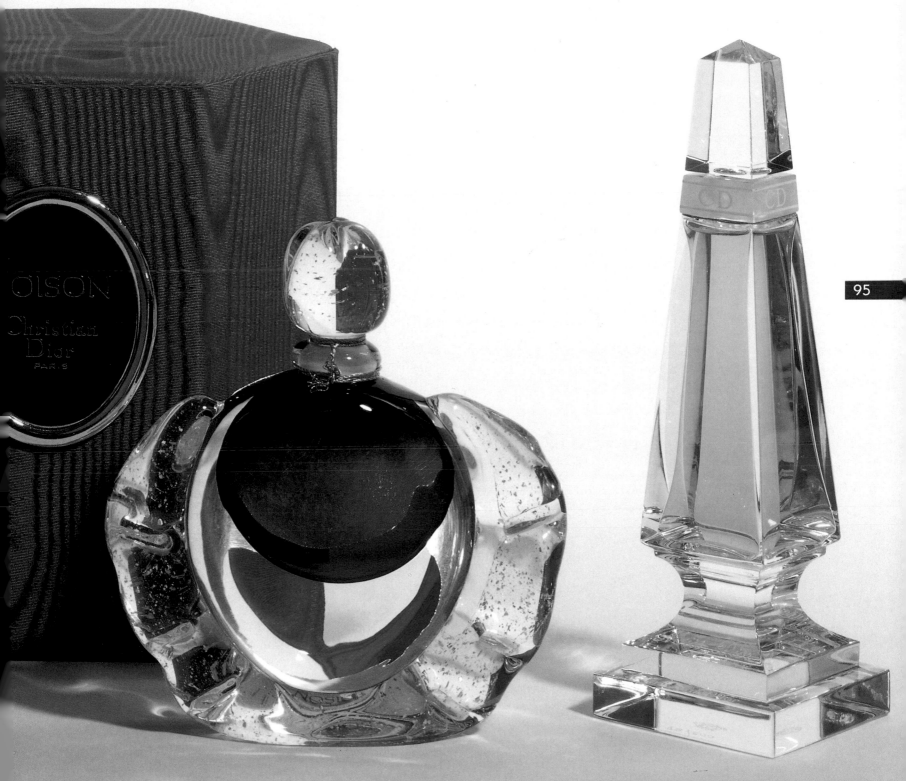

Miss Dior – Christian Dior's first perfume, originally presented in a magnificent Baccarat crystal bottle in the shape of an amphora. In its first year, only two hundred were produced, making it highly sought after by collectors. It was followed by a beautiful design formed by two layers of crystal. The external, colored layer was partially cut to reveal the pure crystal, an effect heightened by the addition of gold. It was produced in the French national colors – red, white and blue – and the design was also used for Diorama in 1948. All the bottles came in superb, classical presention boxes decorated in the grey and white colors of the couturier's studio.

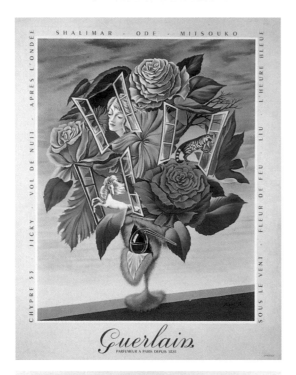

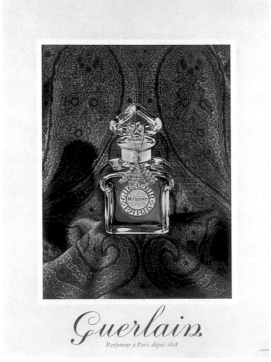

GUERLAIN
A DYNASTY OF PERFUME MAKERS

Pierre-François-Pascal Guerlain was born in Normandy. His father was a craftsman whose violent nature drove the young Guerlain to leave home, travelling first to England, where he trained as a chemist, and later returning to France. In 1828, he opened a shop selling goods imported from England, regarded as the epitome of quality, at 42 rue de Rivoli, on the ground floor of what is today the Hôtel Meurice in Paris. Guerlain soon began to create his own concoctions. The boundaries between *vinaigre*-maker, pharmacist, chemist and perfume-maker were at the time fairly indistinct, and the new company's catalogue featured Canadian bear grease alongside oriental nail polishing powder and skin whitener.

It was, however, specifically as a perfume-distiller that he gained a reputation in fashionable Parisian society. By listening to his customers and mastering perfectly the raw materials at his disposal, Guerlain established the art of blending personalized perfumes, creating an individual eau de toilette for the writer Honoré de Balzac. Yet the strict social convention of the time did not allow for any great originality in perfume-making, discretion being the principle of elegance. Handkerchiefs, fans and camisoles could be scented with small amounts of floral eau de toilette, but the middle class sense of decency dictated that the body remain free from artificial fragrances. In 1840, the house of Guerlain moved to 15 rue de la Paix, in the most fashionable district of Paris, numbering among its clients the Queen of the Belgians and the Prince of Wales. People came from all over Europe to buy perfume from the city's most chic and expensive supplier, and Guerlain's acceptance in the upper echelons of society was confirmed when *Eau de Cologne Impériale*, created for the Empress Eugénie, earned him the honor of Napoleon III's royal warrant.

When he died in 1864, his dual role of managing director and perfume-creator was divided between his sons, Gabriel and Aimé, with the elder Aimé taking over the creation of new fragrances. The restraint that society women were obliged to show in matters of perfume, where the merest hint of an animal note would lead to ostracism on the grounds of poor taste, was gradually abandoned. *Fleur d'Italie* (1884), *Skiné* (1885) and *Rococo* (1887) were perfumes that signalled the emergence of a more artistic approach. However, it was with *Jicky* (1889) that Aimé Guerlain propelled perfumery into the modern era. Far from imitating nature and reproducing the different floral scents of a bouquet, *Jicky* used its animal notes of civet and the addition of the synthetic products coumarin, vanillin and linalol to temper the natural fragrances of lavender and bergamot. As words fail to provide an accurate description of a perfume, *Jicky* was dubbed "original." But success came only with time, over twenty years later.

After *Jicky*, Aimé created *Excellence* in 1890, *Belle-France* in 1892 and *Cipricime* in 1894. Twelve months later, his nephew Jacques (whose nickname was in fact Jicky) succeeded him, creating *Jardin de Mon Curé*, and subsequent years saw the regular launch of new fragrances. The Guerlain catalogue expanded under Jacques's leadership with two or three new products each year. A kind of artistic direction began to evolve, as bottles, labels and graphics were designed to reflect the character of a perfume: in 1900, there was *Voilà Pourquoi J'Aimais Rosine*, with an amazing bouquet of silk begonias decorating its stopper; in 1904, *Champs-Élysées*, with its faceted, tortoise-shaped bottle produced by Baccarat. *Après l'Ondée*, which is still made by Guerlain, was composed in 1906 around a nostalgic, floral blend of violets and hawthorn blossom. *L'Heure Bleue*, created in 1912, another perfume that successfully challenged the tastes of the day, has since become a classic – vivid top notes of Bulgarian rose, orris and heliotrope give way to bewitching, nocturnal middle notes of vanilla, jasmine and musk.

Having moved to the prestigious Champs-Élysées in 1914, the house of Guerlain captured the spirit of the roaring Twenties with similar acuity. Based around a fruity chypre blend celebrating oriental myth, sensuality and reason, *Mitsouko,* created in 1919, is worthy of its name, which in Japanese means "mystery." *Shalimar* (1925) inhabits the same world of oriental delights, but vanilla, frankincense and balsamic notes lend it a more obviously seductive warmth and presence. In 1933, Jacques Guerlain created another exceptional composition with *Vol de Nuit*, whose spirited green and woody dominant notes are softened by vanilla and orris. Taking its inspiration from Hélène Boucher, the famous aviator of the time, it was a perfume for the woman of action, who could succeed in a man's world without losing any of her femininity. Since 1956, Jacques's grandson Jean-Paul has been responsible for creating Guerlain perfumes. The name of his most recent creation, *Héritage* (1992), epitomizes both his own position in the line of succession and the principles which he must uphold – respect for a tradition of quality and sophistication coupled with a constant striving for innovation. "Make good products and never compromise on quality... rely on simple ideas and adhere to them scrupulously": the words of Pierre-François Guerlain have remained guiding principles for the company. The qualities which have earned Guerlain a place in the history of great perfume continue to this day with the daring brilliance of *Chamade* (1969), the confident elegance of *Parure* (1975), the cheerful vivacity of Les *Jardins de Bagatelle* (1983) and the sensual harmony of *Samsara* (1989). These qualities have made Guerlain perfumes timeless, spanning decades and sometimes even centuries, and ensure the longevity of a remarkable company whose research laboratory is today at the forefront of new exciting technology.

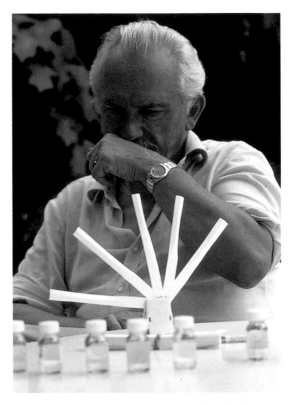

Jean-Paul Guerlain is the latest to follow in the tradition of this great family of perfume-makers.

97

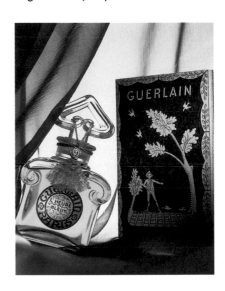

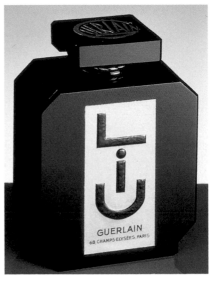

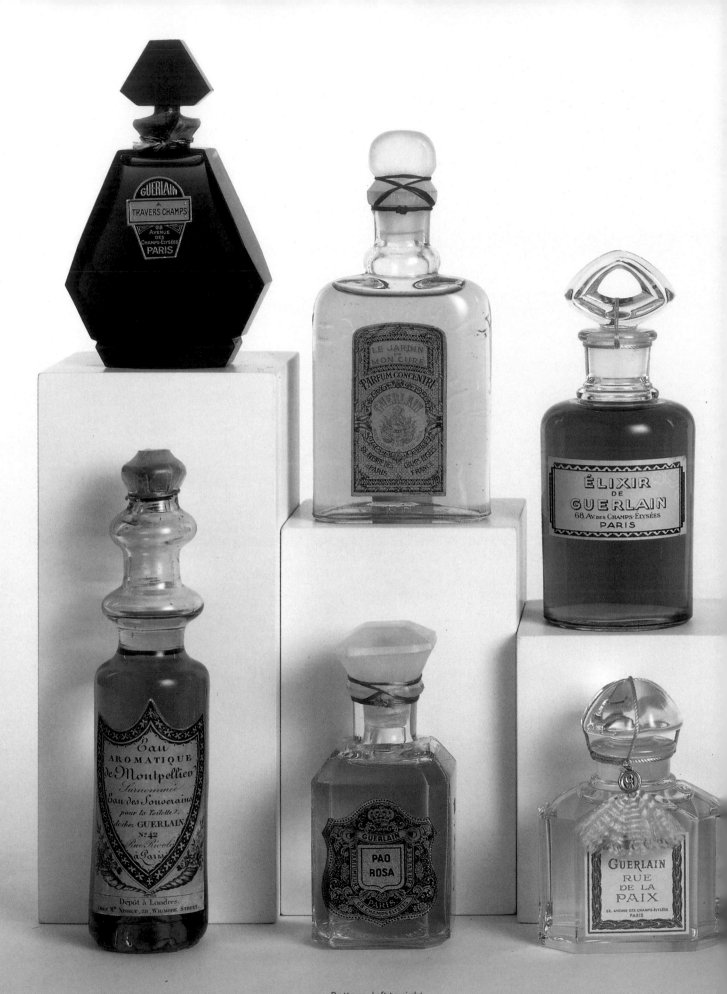

Top, left to right:
À Travers Champs (1924).
Le Jardin de Mon Curé (1895), Jacques Guerlain's first perfume.
Élixir.

Bottom, left to right:
Eau Aromatique de Montpellier.
Pao Rosa.
Rue de la Paix (1908), created to mark the company's return to
this major Parisian thoroughfare.

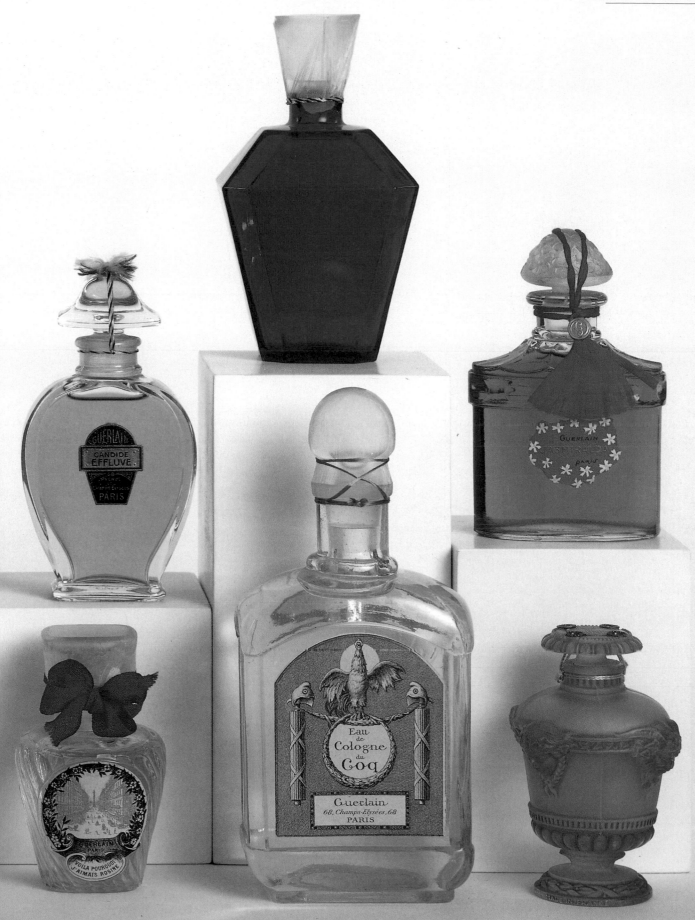

Top, left to right:
Candide Effluve (1924).
Vol de Nuit (1933), created in honor of Saint-Exupéry and here contained in the blue glass bottle also used for other Guerlain fragrances.
Jasmiralda (1917).

Bottom, left to right:
Voilà Pourquoi J'Aimais Rosine (1900), created by Jacques Guerlain for the World Fair in Paris. The vase-shaped bottle was originally topped with a bouquet of silk begonias.
Eau de Cologne du Coq (1894), still sold today.
Bouquet de Faunes (1922).

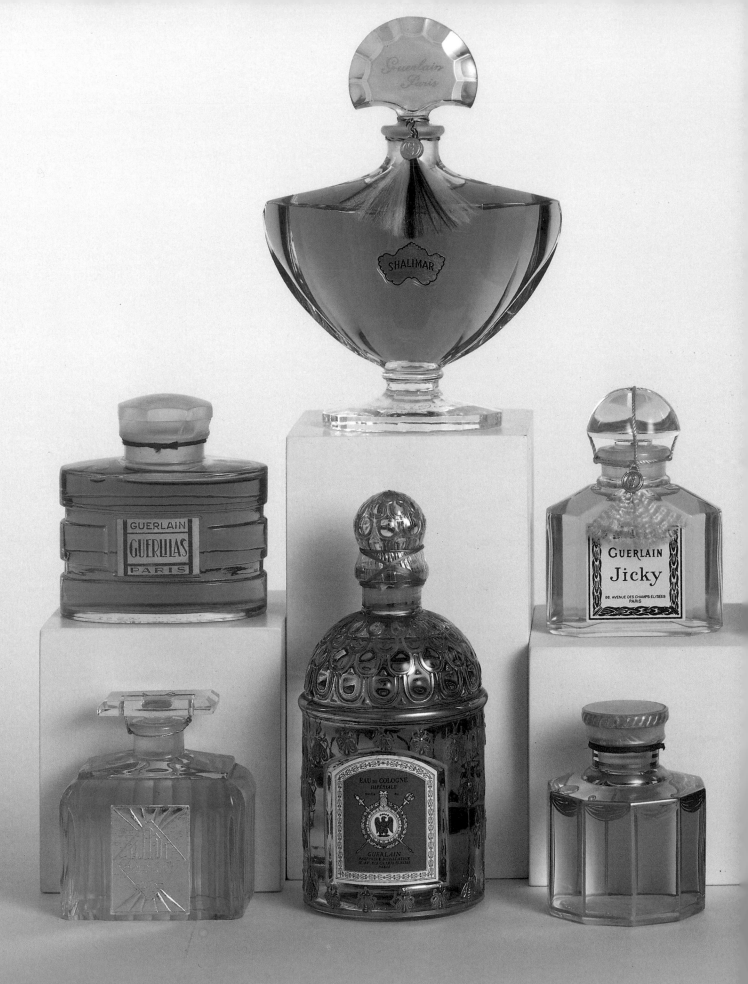

Top, left to right:
Guerlilas *(1930).*
Shalimar *(1925), created by Jacques Guerlain and still sold today.*
Jicky *(1889), aromatic semi-Oriental perfume created by Aimé Guerlain.*

Bottom, left to right:
Djedi *(1927).*
Eau de Cologne Impériale *(1860), created by Pierre-François-Pascal Guerlain for the Empress Eugénie.*
Après l'Ondée *(1906).*

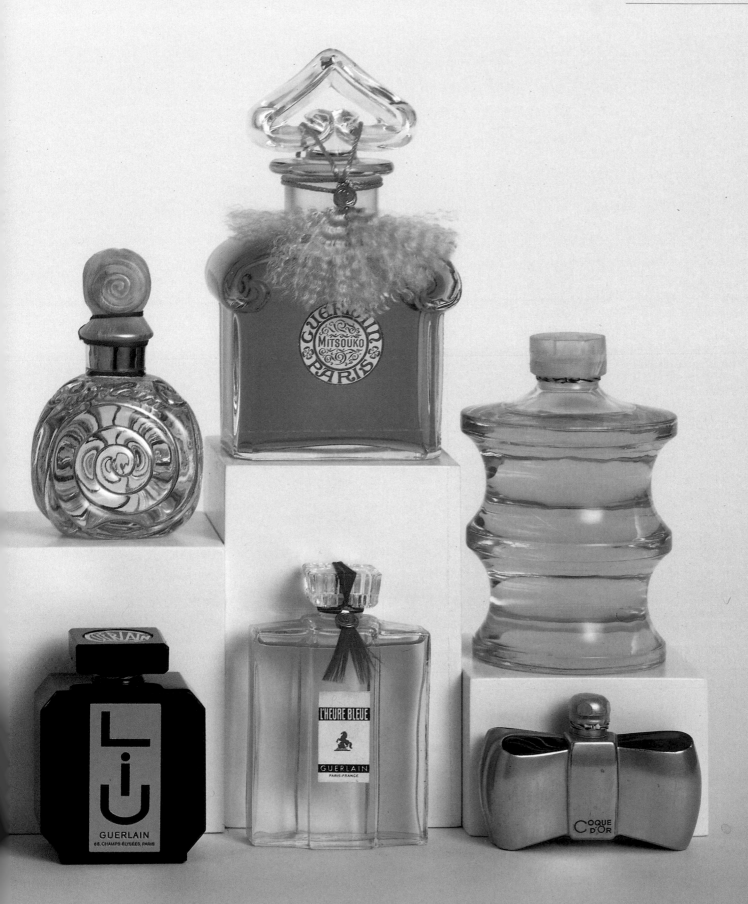

Top, left to right:
Mouchoir de Monsieur *(1904).*
Mitsouko *(1919), a fruity chypre perfume created by
Jacques Guerlain.*
Sous le Vent *(1933).*

Bottom, left to right:
Liu *(1929), recently re-launched.*
L'Heure Bleue *(1912), a flowery semi-Oriental perfume created by
Jacques Guerlain, here in a bottle which is no longer available.*
Coque d'Or *(1937), Baccarat bottle.*

JEANNE LANVIN
THE LADY OF COUTURE

As a girl of thirteen, little Jenny Lanvin wanted to earn her gold louis coin as quickly as possible. Laden with huge hat boxes, she would travel the streets of Paris from dawn to dusk, running behind buses rather than getting on them so as to cut the cost of her errands. Once she had finished making her deliveries, she would go home to her dolls – not to play with them, like other children of her age, but to dress them. She had an extraordinary gift for reproducing dresses in tiny detail on miniature bodies, allowing couturiers to circulate their designs elsewhere in France and abroad. In 1883, at the age of sixteen, she got a job at a milliner's studio and soon rose from apprentice to chief hat-dresser. By 1885, having earned her gold louis, she set up her own business. After three months, the little maid's room on the rue du Marché-Saint-Honoré could no longer cope with the volume of orders and she moved to the rue Saint-Honoré. Within another few months, the studio had moved to the rue des Mathurins and Lanvin allowed herself the luxury of a tricycle, which she used to make her deliveries. When she settled in the rue Boissy-d'Anglas four years later, she had already acquired a reputation as a skillful designer. One day while in Longchamp to observe the polite society who made up her clientele, she met Count Emilio di Pietro – a young, elegant gentleman, albeit avid racegoer and gambler, who set about seducing the young woman. He succeeded, but marriage soon proved too great a sacrifice for such a womanizer. They had a daughter, Marguerite, around whom the rest of Jeanne's life would revolve, but the couple divorced a few years later and Lanvin took refuge in her work. She was an accomplished, exacting businesswoman and the creator of a pure, restrained and unfussy style, who could not resist dressing Marguerite in her own designs. Her customers were enraptured by the little girl with curly blond hair, wanting similar clothes for their own children – the Lanvin children's line was born and clients remained faithful for life.

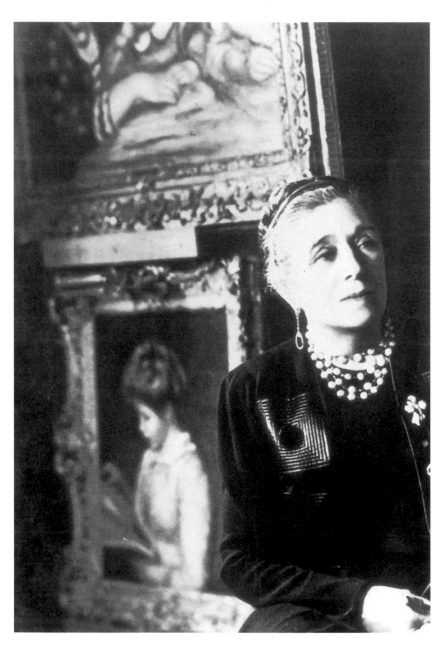

Jeanne Lanvin photographed in the living room of her house on the rue Barbet-de-Jouy, Paris. The interior decoration was by Armand Rateau, who also created the famous, round black bottle for Arpège.
The couturier was a great art lover and on the wall are two beautiful paintings by Renoir.

Jeanne, meanwhile, had already entered the history books and in 1926 was awarded the Légion d'honneur, presented to her by her friend Sacha Guitry. For besides her talents as a designer, "Madame," as she was known, was an art lover and collected paintings by artists such as Renoir, Vuillard and Fantin-Latour. In 1907, she married Xavier Melet, a journalist who later became the French consul in Manchester. She travelled the world with him, taking great pleasure in visiting museums and returning from her trips with sumptuous materials which she kept in what she called her "fabric library." It was during one of her visits to Italy that she was filled with admiration for the blue of a painting by Fra Angelico, the rather mauvish shade which was to become the Lanvin blue. In the meantime, Marguerite had quietly grown up, developing a passion for music and singing. She became Marie-Blanche, Countess de Polignac, by marriage and established herself as a leading figure in the arts. In 1925, Lanvin branched out into perfume, producing fourteen fragrances over the next two years, including *Irisé,* with its subtle trail of violet and orris, *Kara-Djenoun,* inspired by a trip to Egypt, *Géranium d'Espagne, Où Fleurit l'Oranger, Chypre* and *My Sin.* However, the grande dame of couture was still not entirely satisfied and secured the services of André Fraysse, a talented young perfume-blender. She asked him quite simply for "a unique and timeless masterpiece," with her only instructions being, "Think of Marie-Blanche." The masterpiece was created in 1927, a harmonious mix of Bulgarian rose and Grasse jasmine, subtly blended with mock orange, lily of the valley and honeysuckle. With over sixty floral notes, this superb blend was difficult to name, but when Marie-Blanche took a sniff from the test strip, one word sprang to her mind: *Arpège.*

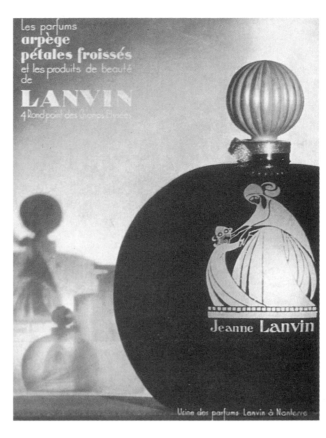

*"I am concerned with perfection, not budgets or fashion."
With these words, Jeanne Lanvin commissioned* Arpège
from the perfume-blender André Fraysse.

103

The perfume demanded an exceptional bottle, and one which broke with the styles of the time. Lanvin commissioned its design from Armand Rateau, the well-known sculptor and decorator to whom she had entrusted the interior design of her house. He created the famous black ball, with fine gold decoration by the designer Paul Iribe. Again it was Marie-Blanche who provided the inspiration for what is still the company logo today: mother and daughter are in evening dress and Jeanne leans towards Marie-Blanche with outstretched arms. The famous black spheres, perfect examples of art deco styling, would later be used for other company perfumes. In 1928, Lanvin launched *Âme Perdue* and *Pétales Froissés,* followed in subsequent years by *Scandal, Eau de Lanvin, Eau de Cologne, Rumeur* and finally *Prétexte.* All these compositions reflected the refinement, reserve and perfectionism of the woman whom the English dubbed "the lady of couture." When she died, in July 1946, it was Marie-Blanche who this time leaned towards her mother to slip into her hand the gold louis which she had earned with such perseverance sixty years earlier.

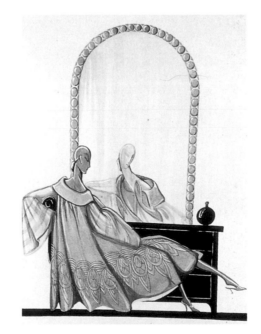

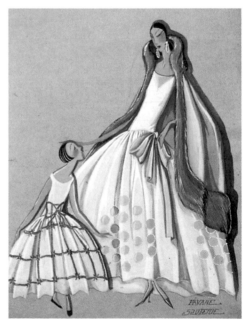

Jeanne Lanvin made her mark on twentieth-century fashion with a restrained, harmonious style that emphasized feminine grace. She hated easy, mannered effects and avoided using any detail which might date a dress, resulting in timeless clothes in subtle shades and of delightful simplicity.

The famous ball, designed in 1927, is the work of two artists: Armand Rateau, Jeanne Lanvin's favorite decorator; and Paul Iribe, designer of the figure which today is still the company logo.

The bottles are highly sought after by collectors and come in a range of different sizes and colors – black, gold, crystal and the very rare Sèvres porcelain examples, produced in numbered limited editions and in blue, turquoise or purple. They were made to order and contained extracts of Lanvin's leading perfumes – Lajea, La Dogaresse, My Sin, Chypre, Comme Ci Comme Ça, J'En Raffole and later, the most famous of all, Arpège.

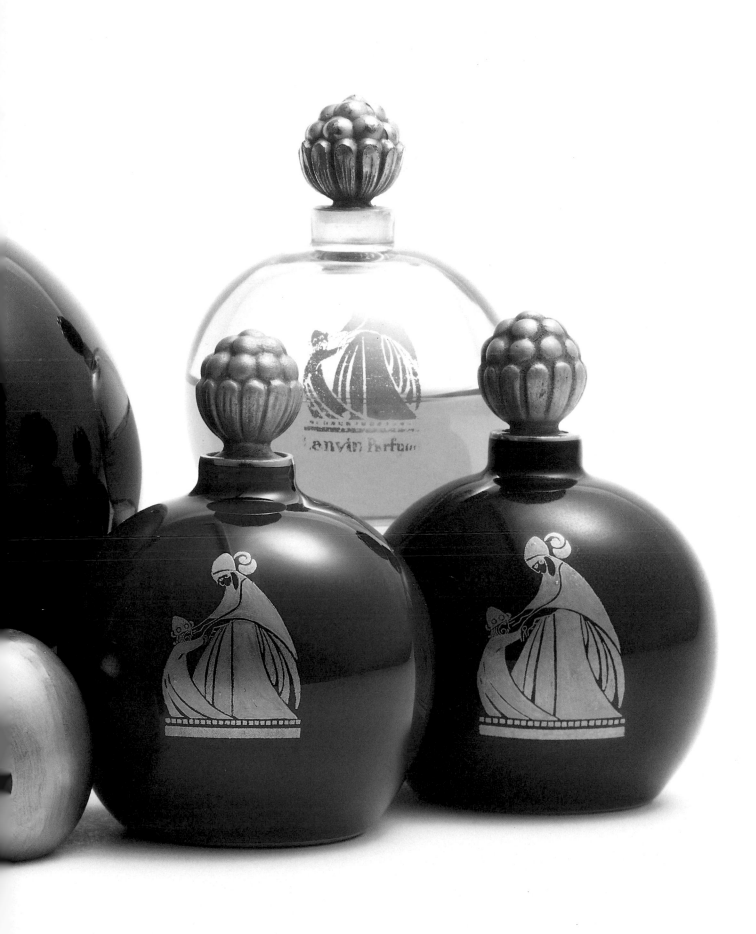

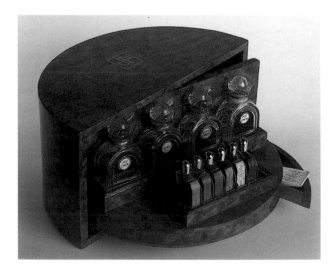

SUBLIME...

JEAN PATOU

Sublime, Patou's most recent perfume for women. In keeping with tradition, the great Parisian company used the most precious raw materials to compose this flowery semi-Oriental fragrance – rose, jasmine and lily of the valley, blended with orange flower, vetiver, sandalwood and oak moss.

Patou built a bar, decorated in the cubist style, on the ground floor of his house on the rue Saint-Florentin. Here, his clients could sample a number of essences and ask the bartender to blend perfumes for them, just like a cocktail. The bar was designed by the architects Louis Süe and André Mare, who were also responsible for the interior design of Patou's head office.
Below: *Miniature version of the bar with its various samples.*

JEAN PATOU
THE ESSENCE OF FASHION

Having served in the army during some of the fiercest fighting on the Dardanelles front in 1915, Jean Patou knew the hardships, fear and horror of battle. Returning to Paris to resume the career of couturier which he had begun before the war, this handsome son of a wealthy leather-tanning family soon understood that these experiences would shape the rest of his life. The restless and rather frivolous pre-war young man had disappeared in favor of a determined entrepreneur, with very specific ideas on the simple styles he wanted to create and something of a taste for the thrills of gambling and risk-taking. Patou knew that he had lost many of his former customers – some had deserted him for Coco Chanel, whose designs won her a huge following. Soon grasping the importance of creating his own niche in the market, he left Chanel with her clientele – stemming from the intelligentsia and the arts, with traditional tastes but open to modernist ideas – and targeted high society. He understood perfectly the needs of a class undergoing complete transformation as it divided its time between the most fashionable places in the world – Paris, New York, the palaces of the Riviera, ski resorts and so on. With the help of an unparalleled team of colleagues, he would inject the spirit of the Twenties into fashion and become the symbol of the carefree inter-war generation.

As the designer of co-ordinating knitwear and instigator of sportswear for women such as the famous blue and white-striped sweaters worn over pleated skirts, he enjoyed rapid success in the United States. He was also the first couturier to accessorize his clothes with bags and hats, which he called "little nothings," and to use his monogram as a stylistic device. He was later to engineer a pivotal moment in Parisian haute couture by his daring use of American catwalk models, whose figures differed from those of French women. When she appeared at Wimbledon in 1921, dressed in a pleated silk knee-length skirt, sleeveless white cardigan and orange headband, the great tennis player Suzanne Lenglen created a sensation. She was an excellent ambassador for Patou's fashions, and this image of the athletic but clothes-conscious woman would serve him well. His love of women was well-known and, although he never married, he is said to have had many affairs. It should come as no surprise, therefore, that his first perfumes, launched in 1925, should have names which evoke the different stages of love – *Amour-Amour, Que Sais-Je?* and *Adieu Sagesse*. All three compositions featured fruity, floral notes which Patou had created for what he regarded as the three main types of women: *Amour-Amour* was a heady fragrance designed for sensual brunettes; the lighter *Que Sais-Je?* was intended for blondes; while *Adieu Sagesse*, with its overtly spicy accents, was reserved exclusively for redheads. Four years later, Patou launched the innovative *Le Sien*, the first unisex perfume. He had wanted, "... a fresh, invigorating perfume with dominant masculine notes, perfectly suited to men, but also to resolutely modern women who play golf, smoke and drive fast cars." The same year, the launch of *Moment Suprême* coincided with the New York stock market collapse. All the bottles, which were fitted with pineapple-shaped stoppers, were designed by Louis Süe and André Mare, two architects and decorators to whom Patou had also entrusted the interior design of his own house. However, the company still lacked a "signature" perfume, like Chanel's recently created *No.5*. In early 1930, Patou went to Grasse, accompanied by his friend and advisor Elsa Maxwell, with the aim of creating a unique and luxurious perfume that would have immediate commercial success. This was no easy task, as Elsa Maxwell recalls in her memoirs, "We had tried everything ... all that Almeras, Patou's in-house perfume-blender, had suggested to us, but nothing matched what we were looking for. In despair, and on the point of giving up, he showed us one last perfume, composed with the most precious essences of rose and jasmine." As soon as he had done so, Henri Almeras added that the production costs of the blend were far too high for it to be commercially viable. He had failed to take Patou's sense of daring into account, for the designer was immediately smitten with the idea of using the richest products in the same way that the most beautiful fabrics are used in haute couture. Elsa Maxwell, whose forceful personality was familiar to Parisian high society, devised its slogan: *"Joy*, the costliest perfume in the world." Patou understood his clientele and knew that he could justify such an advertisement even at the height of the Depression. Over sixty years after its creation, *Joy* remains one of the five best-selling perfumes in the world and is still made using the most beautiful jasmine flowers and the best Grasse roses.

In 1933, Patou launched *Divine Folie*, followed in 1935 by *Normandie*, which was given to every passenger on the famous liner's maiden voyage. Their success led to a continued use of symbolism and he produced *Vacances* to mark the introduction of paid holidays. It was to be his last creation, for he died prematurely in 1936. His brother-in-law, Raymond Barbas, took over and created new perfumes in the same tradition: *Colony*, launched in 1938 when dreams of fleeing overseas pervaded pre-war Europe; *L'Heure Attendue* in 1946 to celebrate the Liberation; and *Câline* in 1964. These were followed by *1,000* (1972), like *Joy*, a perfume composed of extremely precious essences, *Eau de Patou* (1976), *Patou Pour Homme* (1980) and *Sublime* (1992). All these were created by Jean Kerléo, Patou's blender since 1967, who produces the fragrances himself in his laboratory at the Patou factory. The memory of Jean Patou, a man obsessed with quality and innovation, remains the company's guiding principle.

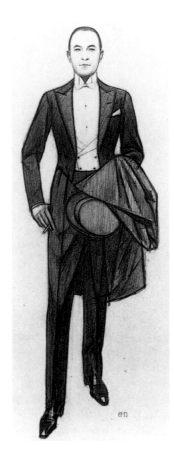

"A sophisticated woman should avoid all eccentricity, in the choice of a perfume as much as in that of a dress, applying the same discreet sense of taste and elegance to her scent as to her wardrobe." With these words, Patou addressed his clients until his untimely death in 1936.

107

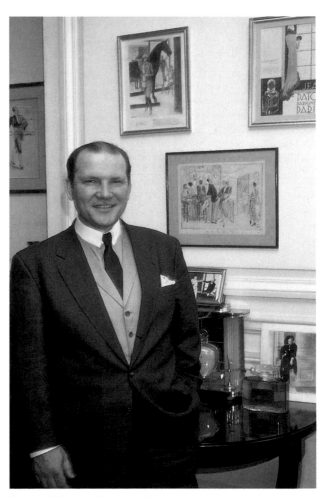

Since 1980, the House of Patou's managing director has been Jean de Moüy, the couturier's great-great-nephew.

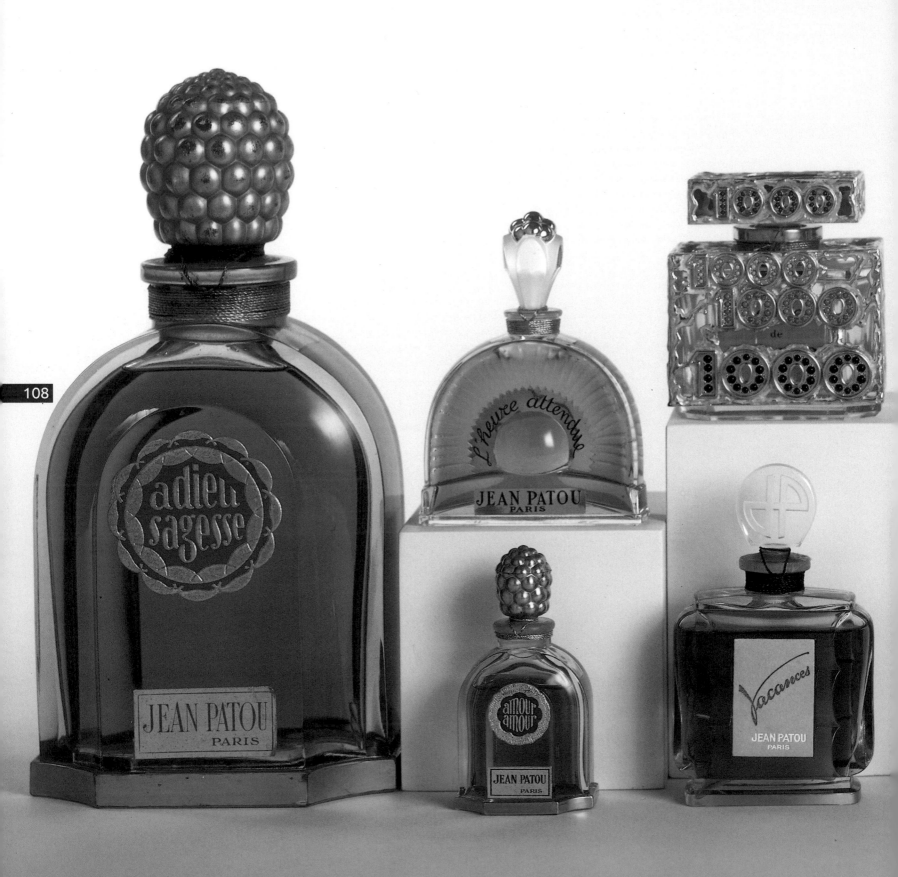

108

Top, left to right:
Adieu Sagesse *(1925), one of Patou's early perfumes.*
L'Heure Attendue *(1946), created to celebrate the Liberation.*
The bottle was reproduced in 1991 in a limited edition of 350.
1,000 *(1972), limited edition bottle made by jewellers.*

Bottom, left to right:
Amour-Amour *(1925), Patou's first perfume.*
Vacances *(1936), launched to mark the introduction of*
paid holidays.

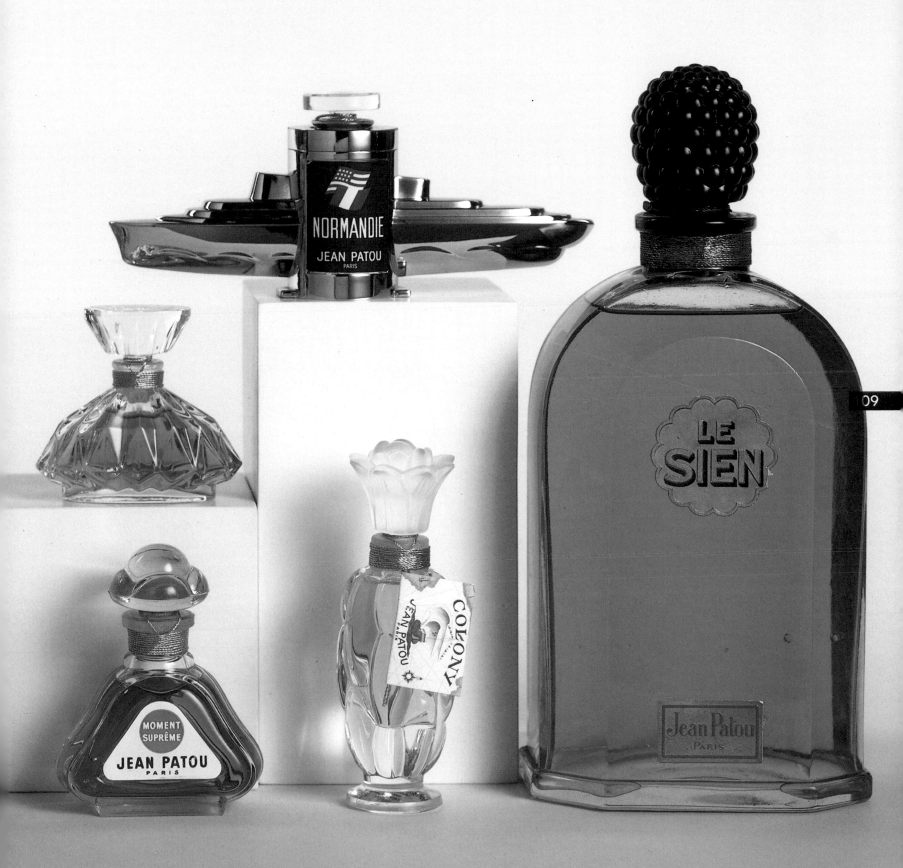

Top, left to right:
Joy *(1930)*, Baccarat bottle dating from 1975 and still
sold today.
Normandie *(1935)*, created to mark the liner's maiden
voyage. The bottle was reproduced in 1989 in a limited
edition of 1,000.
Le Sien *(1929)*, the first unisex perfume.

Bottom, left to right:
Moment Suprême *(1929)*.
Colony *(1938)*, original "pineapple" bottle design reproduced in
1994 in a limited edition of 1,000.

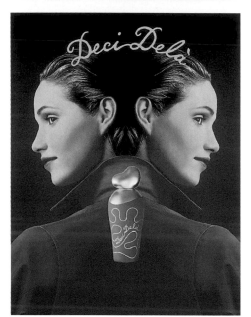

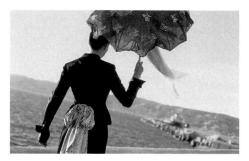

Above: *Through its fashions and its perfumes, Nina Ricci today remains a paragon of French haute couture. Its most recent fragrance, Deci Delà, was launched in 1994 to great acclaim.*

Below: *The Nina Ricci perfume factory at Ury. Robert Ricci took a great interest in the quality of the environment in which his employees would develop.*

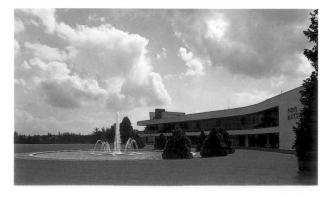

NINA RICCI
TIMELESS ROMANTICISM

When, as a child growing up near Turin, Marie Adelaide Nielli was making eye-catching hats trimmed with tiny decorations for her relatives, she was unaware that she would become one of twentieth-century fashion's most important figures. It was, however, natural that she should turn toward couture, first working as a seamstress and later as an appointed designer. At the age of eighteen, she was head of a studio and married Louis Ricci, moving to Monte Carlo and then Paris, where she became a designer. By 1905, when she gave birth to her son Robert, she was creating her own designs for major labels.

In 1932, having already acquired an international reputation, she decided to open her own haute couture business, which was to be called "Nina Ricci" and would be managed by her son, Robert. Her studio, at 20 rue des Capucines, in Paris, was always full and Madame Ricci's female clientele appreciated the subtle charm and sophistication of her designs. She was more of an architect than a draftsman, adapting her designs to the individual personalities of her clients. Her perfect understanding of couture, coupled with a superb mastery of cutting (which she did herself by draping the fabric directly over a dummy), made her style one of the most original and fresh of the pre-war period. Just before the outbreak of the Second World War, Nina Ricci occupied three buildings and eleven floors on the rue des Capucines. In 1950, on the advice of her son, Madame Ricci decided to employ young designers and so it was that Jules-François Crahay joined the company and soon enjoyed great success. He was succeeded in 1964 by Gérard Pipart, who is still in charge of the haute couture studio and received the profession's twenty-second Golden Thimble award.

In 1946, concerned with the diversification of the company's activities and the expression of its character, Robert Ricci gave it a new dimension by creating a perfume. Research, quality and respect for women were the driving forces behind his inspiration. With the help of perfume-blenders, he produced an aldehydic floral fragrance named *Cœur-Joie*, commissioning its bottle from his childhood friend, Marc Lalique. Their success was immediate and reinforced two years later with the launch of a second perfume, *L'Air du Temps*, which has since become one of the classics of perfumery. Its bottle, also by Marc Lalique with flowers designed by the painter Christian Bérard, is recognized all over the world – the two doves on the stopper are a symbol of both peace and eternal youth. Today, on average, a bottle of *L'Air du Temps* is sold somewhere in the world every second. According to Robert Ricci, perfume should idealize a woman – "We must serve a woman without using her" was a phrase which he was fond of repeating. Throughout his life, he was a fierce defender of the creative process, as can be seen in the quality of his perfumes, of course, but also in the beauty of the bottles and their boxes and even in the artistic aspects of their advertising material. Thus, the painter Christian Bérard worked on the bottle for *Cœur-Joie*, while Andy Warhol and David Hamilton contributed to the worldwide promotion of the company image. In his capacity as blender, Robert Ricci was involved in the creation of all the perfumes, making the final decision himself without resorting to the battery of tests so beloved of large companies' marketing departments. Although today such an approach might seem more difficult to undertake, or at least a great deal more risky, it allowed this great company to secure its place in the history of perfume.

The partnership with Lalique produced seven sumptuous bottles created by the great crystal-maker – *Cœur-Joie* (1946), *L'Air du Temps* (1951), *Fille d'Ève* (1952), *Capricci* (1961), *Farouche* (1974), *Fleur de Fleur* (1982) and *Nina* (1987). They are highly prized by collectors and are made at Wingen-sur-Moder in Alsace, which has been the home of the crystal works since 1920. Each piece, produced using traditional techniques, undergoes about fifteen stages of finishing, carried out manually by craftsmen, including polishing, cutting, satining with sand to obtain the required degree of transparency and grinding the stopper. Since 1973, the perfumes themselves have been produced and packaged at Ury, south of Paris, in a factory where traditional skill is combined with state of the art technology. Here, Robert Ricci took a great interest in creating working conditions and an environment in which his workers could thrive and develop. He chose the trees and flowers planted in the large garden surrounding the factory and supervised the construction of modern, well-lit workshops. One hundred thousand bottles are packaged there daily and over twenty-five million products are dispatched worldwide every year.

Today, despite the death of both Madame Ricci and Robert, Nina Ricci remains an independent family company. It is managed by Gilles Fuchs, Robert Ricci's son-in-law, and its products – haute couture, prêt-à-porter collections, fashion accessories, beauty products and, of course, perfume – are sold all over the world. To date, the Nina Ricci range comprises eight perfumes for women and two for men. Just before his death, at the age of eighty-three on August 8, 1988, Robert Ricci paid great homage to his mother with the creation of a beautiful floral perfume which he named simply *Nina*. The most recent addition to the family is called *Deci Delà* and its bottle, by the artists Garouste and Bonetti, recaptures Ricci's characteristic playful and romantic style.

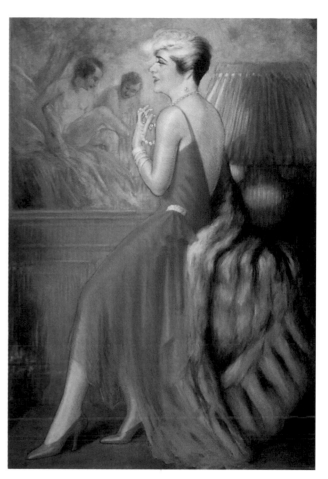

111

Above: "Madame Nina Ricci" painted in 1932 by Cireuse.
Below: Robert Ricci was responsible for the creation of Nina Ricci perfumes and fought to maintain the artistic tradition of French perfumery.

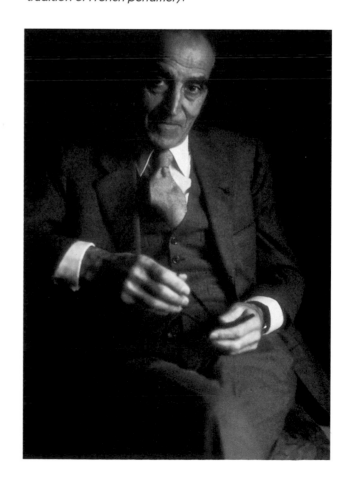

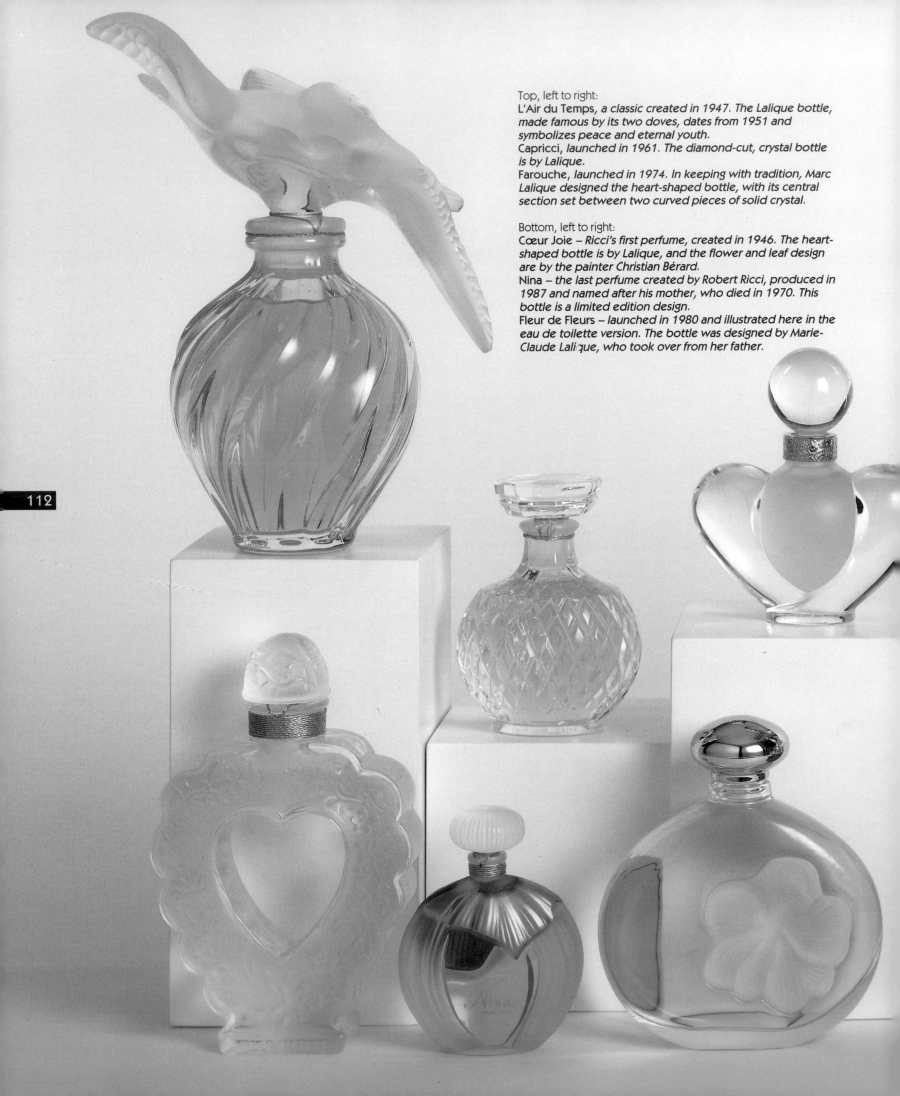

Top, left to right:
L'Air du Temps, a classic created in 1947. The Lalique bottle, made famous by its two doves, dates from 1951 and symbolizes peace and eternal youth.
Capricci, launched in 1961. The diamond-cut, crystal bottle is by Lalique.
Farouche, launched in 1974. In keeping with tradition, Marc Lalique designed the heart-shaped bottle, with its central section set between two curved pieces of solid crystal.

Bottom, left to right:
Cœur Joie – Ricci's first perfume, created in 1946. The heart-shaped bottle is by Lalique, and the flower and leaf design are by the painter Christian Bérard.
Nina – the last perfume created by Robert Ricci, produced in 1987 and named after his mother, who died in 1970. This bottle is a limited edition design.
Fleur de Fleurs – launched in 1980 and illustrated here in the eau de toilette version. The bottle was designed by Marie-Claude Lalique, who took over from her father.

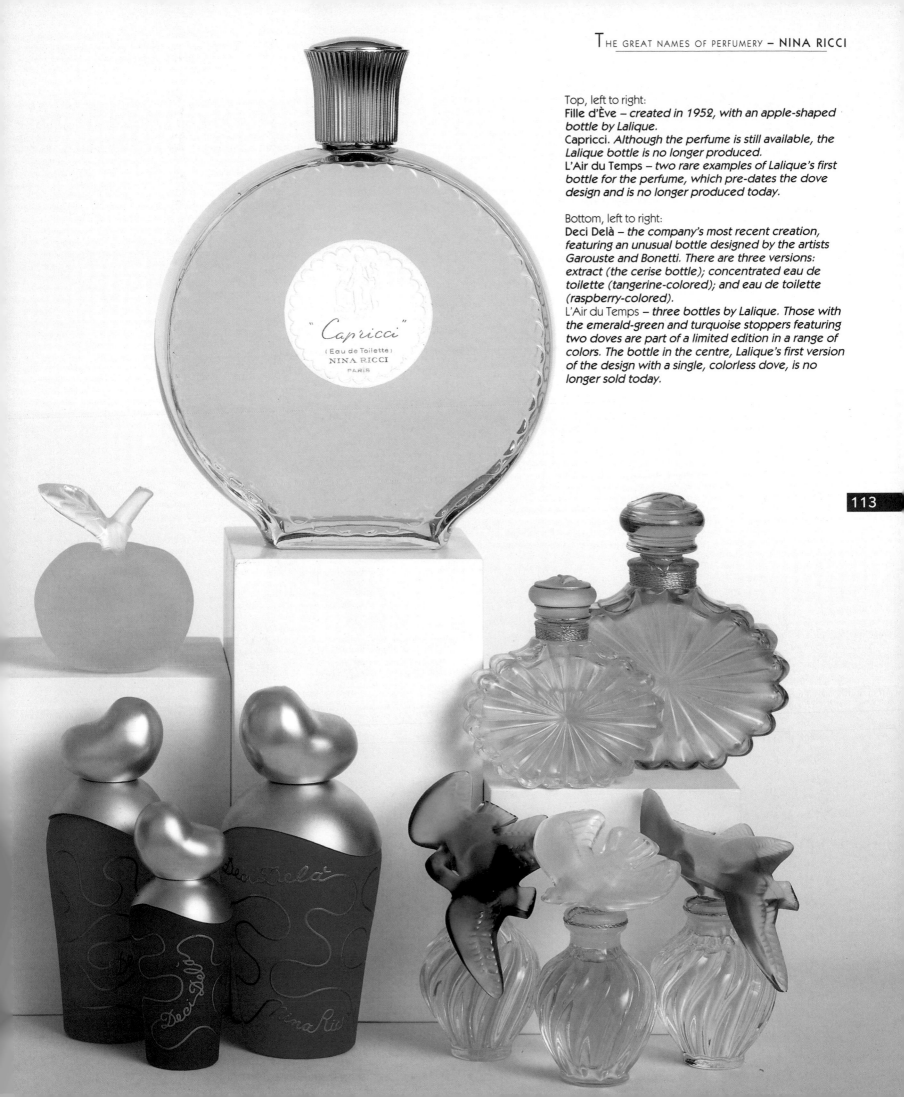

Top, left to right:
Fille d'Ève – *created in 1952, with an apple-shaped bottle by Lalique.*
Capricci. *Although the perfume is still available, the Lalique bottle is no longer produced.*
L'Air du Temps – *two rare examples of Lalique's first bottle for the perfume, which pre-dates the dove design and is no longer produced today.*

Bottom, left to right:
Deci Delà – *the company's most recent creation, featuring an unusual bottle designed by the artists Garouste and Bonetti. There are three versions: extract (the cerise bottle); concentrated eau de toilette (tangerine-colored); and eau de toilette (raspberry-colored).*
L'Air du Temps – *three bottles by Lalique. Those with the emerald-green and turquoise stoppers featuring two doves are part of a limited edition in a range of colors. The bottle in the centre, Lalique's first version of the design with a single, colorless dove, is no longer sold today.*

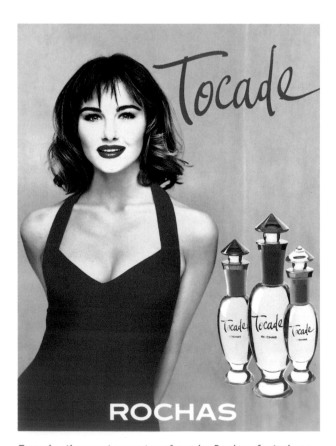

EAU DE ROCHAS

ROCHAS

Typical of the refreshing perfumes in vogue during the Seventies, Eau de Rochas, *with its combined notes of verbena and lime, has retained its attraction.*

Tocade

ROCHAS

Tocade, *the most recent perfume by Rochas, featuring a harmonious blend of rose, vanilla and ambergris.*

ROCHAS
HIS ERA WAS HIS GUIDE

"My era was my guide" – Marcel Rochas' words reflect the essence of his designs. Born in 1902, the man who was to remain best-known as the inventor of the girdle opened his couture business in 1920, in partnership with a Paul Poiret fashion model.

Following the example of his contemporaries Coco Chanel and Jean Patou, Rochas soon overturned the rules of elegance. In 1925, thanks to him, women discovered irreverent and fluid styles which combined grace with a subtlety of touch. He gave them narrow hips, a slender waist and graceful shoulders, using wool like silk, turning lace into a symbol of sensuality and crepe into sculpture. A wing would appear on a shoulder, as it does on the famous black and white piqué evening dress which he designed in 1931. In this thrilling decade which saw the rise of the charleston, the wild Montparnasse nightclub scene, Picasso and Stravinsky, it seemed that nothing could stop the young couturier.

In 1932, he moved to number 12 avenue Matignon, in the heart of what is still Paris's most exclusive shopping district, and *Avenue Matignon* was to be the name of the first Rochas perfume, launched in 1936 at the same time as *Air Jeune* and *Audace.* The couturier was fond of saying that, "One should notice the scent of a woman before even seeing her." He produced a huge range of innovations – the fitted suit, the fur-lined jacket, patterned prints and, most famous of all, the gypsy dress, which was his best-selling design in the United States. It was there that Marcel Rochas found real fame, becoming the darling of film stars – he made Hollywood his second home and dressed screen legends such as Loretta Young, Joan Crawford, Katharine Hepburn, Jean Harlow, Carole Lombard and Marlene Dietrich. His favorite, however, and the one who without any doubt proved his greatest inspiration, was Mae West, for whom he designed an infamously sexy black lace girdle.

In 1943, the perfume-blender Edmond Roudnitska offered Rochas a beautiful, fruity chypre composition which blended peach and plum with white flowers over base notes of musk, ambergris and sandalwood. The couturier was won over and in 1944 launched the perfume on a subscription basis, as wartime rationing severely limited its availability. It was also in this year that Rochas married Hélène, an extraordinary young woman who would play an important role in the company. *Femme,* with its Lalique crystal, amphora-shaped bottle, was dedicated to her and sold only to a limited circle of people: the Duchess of Windsor, Baroness Rothschild, Michèle Morgan, Danielle Darrieux and Arletty were the first to wear the fragrance. The general public had to wait another year before the perfume reached the shops. Its launch was marked by a cocktail party which also paid homage to Paul Poiret, the first couturier to have created a perfume. In 1946, Edmond Roudnitska repeated the success with *Chiffon* and *Poupée*. He remained the Rochas perfume-blender, creating *Mousseline* (1947), *L'Eau de Verveine* (1948), *La Rose* (1949), Marcel Rochas' favorite perfume, and, most famously, *Moustache* (1949). For the first time in the history of men's perfumery, an entire line accompanied the fragrance and an extract for men was produced.

By 1952, Marcel Rochas Perfumes was a thriving company based at Asnières in suburbs of Paris, employing fifty-five staff who ensured the worldwide distribution of just under half a million items. Such was its success that Rochas abandoned dress design and closed his couture house in 1953. Unfortunately, he died prematurely two years later, having only briefly enjoyed his new career. Hélène Rochas took over and in 1960 launched *Madame Rochas*, an aldehydic floral perfume created by Guy Robert. It is a subtle cocktail of flowers, among which jasmine, narcissus and tuberose are the most easily recognizable – Hélène Rochas was a great lover of white flowers and they were included in all the compositions which she commissioned. The bottle for *Madame Rochas* is a replica of an eighteenth-century, Baccarat crystal *janusette* which Hélène had spotted in the window of a Parisian antique shop; its classical design, along with the tapestry cover of its box, sneered at the Sixties art scene. Its Paris launch was marked by a beautiful exhibition at the Galliera, entitled "Portraits of Women," and Parisian high society flocked to the preview to admire works by Picasso, Monet, Matisse and Fragonard. *Madame Rochas* soon became an international success and established Hélène, now managing director, as an accomplished professional. In 1965, she was voted one of the twelve most elegant women in the world and was dubbed "The Perfume Queen."

Guy Robert created *Monsieur Rochas* in 1969, the year which saw the opening of the Poissy factory, a vast, modern ninety-five thousand square foot complex employing three hundred and twenty-five staff. In 1970, Nicolas Mamounas created *Eau de Roche*, later renamed *Eau de Rochas*, a refreshing fragrance for women with base notes of lime and verbena, and went on to produce *Mystère de Rochas* (1978), *Macassar* (1980), for men, and *Lumière* (1984) and *Byzance* (1987), both for women. *Globe* (1990), for men, and *Eau de Rochas Pour Homme* were to follow. *Tocade* (1994), the most recent creation, is a rich fragrance for women based on a blend of rose, vanilla and ambergris. Both *Femme* and *Madame Rochas* have been re-designed, remaining true to the fragrant richness of the originals while borrowing the structure of a modern perfume. A new chapter in the history of Rochas was opened when it was bought in 1987 by the German group Wella, and it seems safe to assume that this great company will meet the challenges of the next century with as much daring innovation as it showed at the start of this one.

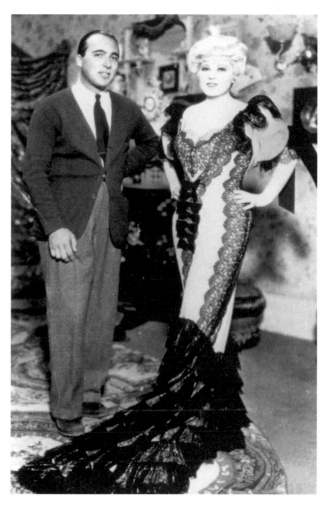

115

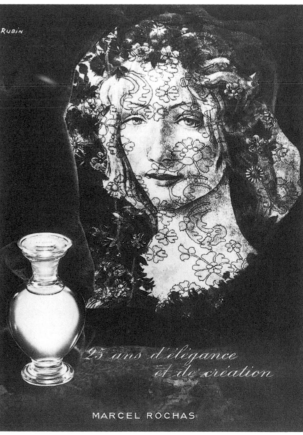

Marcel Rochas with Mae West at the peak of her Hollywood career. The two artists were lifelong friends and legend has it that the bottle for Femme *was inspired by the actress's curvaceous figure.*

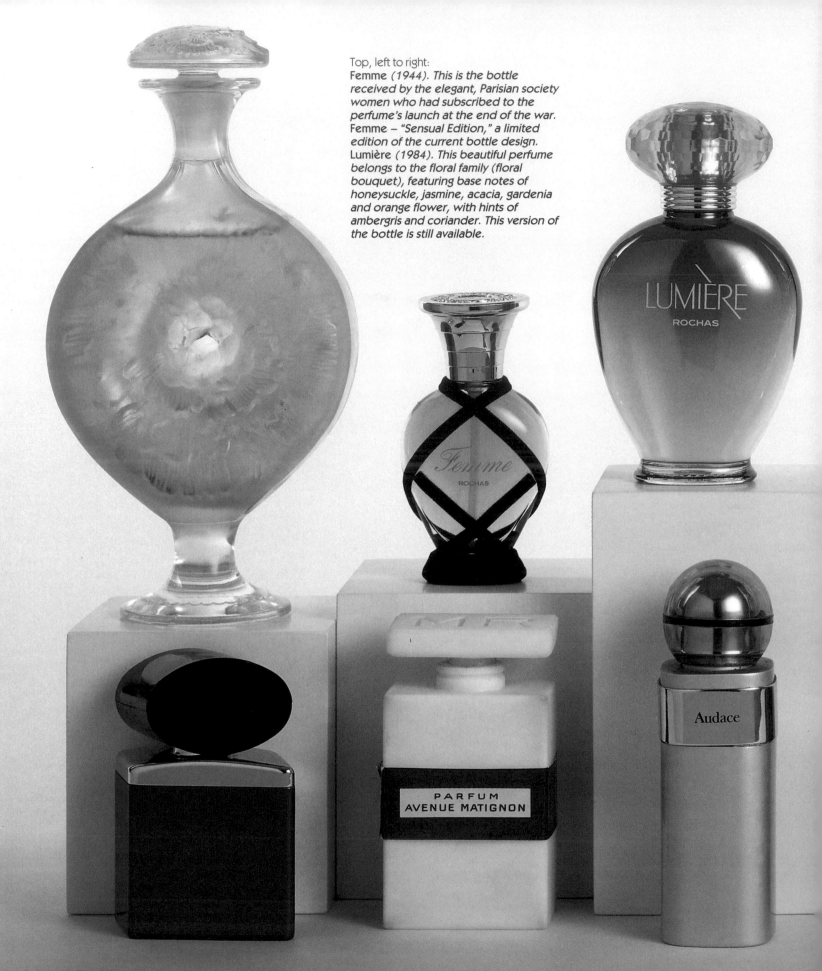

Top, left to right:
Femme *(1944). This is the bottle received by the elegant, Parisian society women who had subscribed to the perfume's launch at the end of the war.*
Femme – "Sensual Edition," *a limited edition of the current bottle design.*
Lumière *(1984). This beautiful perfume belongs to the floral family (floral bouquet), featuring base notes of honeysuckle, jasmine, acacia, gardenia and orange flower, with hints of ambergris and coriander. This version of the bottle is still available.*

Bottom, left to right:
Mystère de Rochas *(1978). The perfume belongs to the chypre family (aldehydic flowery chypre), featuring base notes of bergamot, honeysuckle, jasmine, rose, narcissus, gardenia, magnolia, ylang-ylang, mosses and precious woods. This atomizer is no longer available.*
Avenue Matignon *– Rochas' first perfume, which took its name from the first couture house opened by Marcel Rochas in 1920. The shape of the bottle recalls that of another, very famous fragrance.*
Audace *(1971). An earlier perfume of the same name had been created in 1936. This blend, totally different from the first, was taken off the market in 1978.*

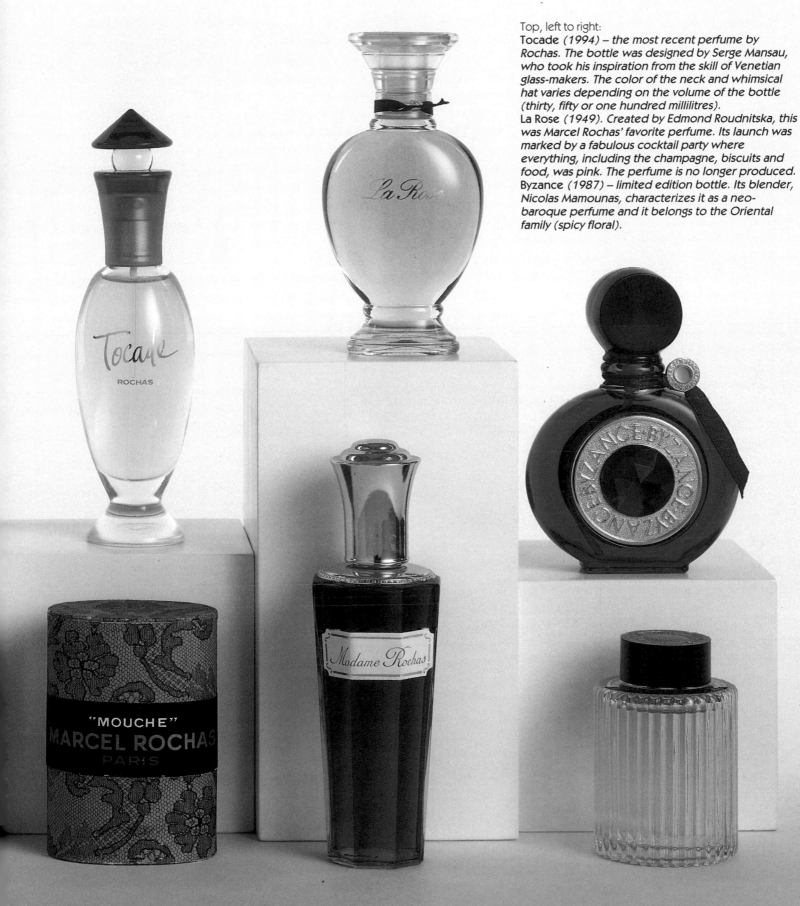

Top, left to right:

Tocade (1994) – the most recent perfume by Rochas. The bottle was designed by Serge Mansau, who took his inspiration from the skill of Venetian glass-makers. The color of the neck and whimsical hat varies depending on the volume of the bottle (thirty, fifty or one hundred millilitres).

La Rose (1949). Created by Edmond Roudnitska, this was Marcel Rochas' favorite perfume. Its launch was marked by a fabulous cocktail party where everything, including the champagne, biscuits and food, was pink. The perfume is no longer produced.

Byzance (1987) – limited edition bottle. Its blender, Nicolas Mamounas, characterizes it as a neo-baroque perfume and it belongs to the Oriental family (spicy floral).

Bottom, left to right:

Mouche (1948). This winter perfume, created to be worn on furs, was composed of musk, opopanax and ambergris. The bottle took the traditional shape of Rochas perfume-bottles (identical to Femme and La Rose).

Madame Rochas (1960) – the first perfume launched by Hélène Rochas after her husband's death. It belongs to the floral family (aldehydic floral) and the bottle is still available.

Moustache (1949) – eau de toilette for men created by Edmond Roudnitska, now no longer produced. It was the first perfume to be accompanied by a complete line of products (aftershave, toiletries, etc.), including the first extract for men.

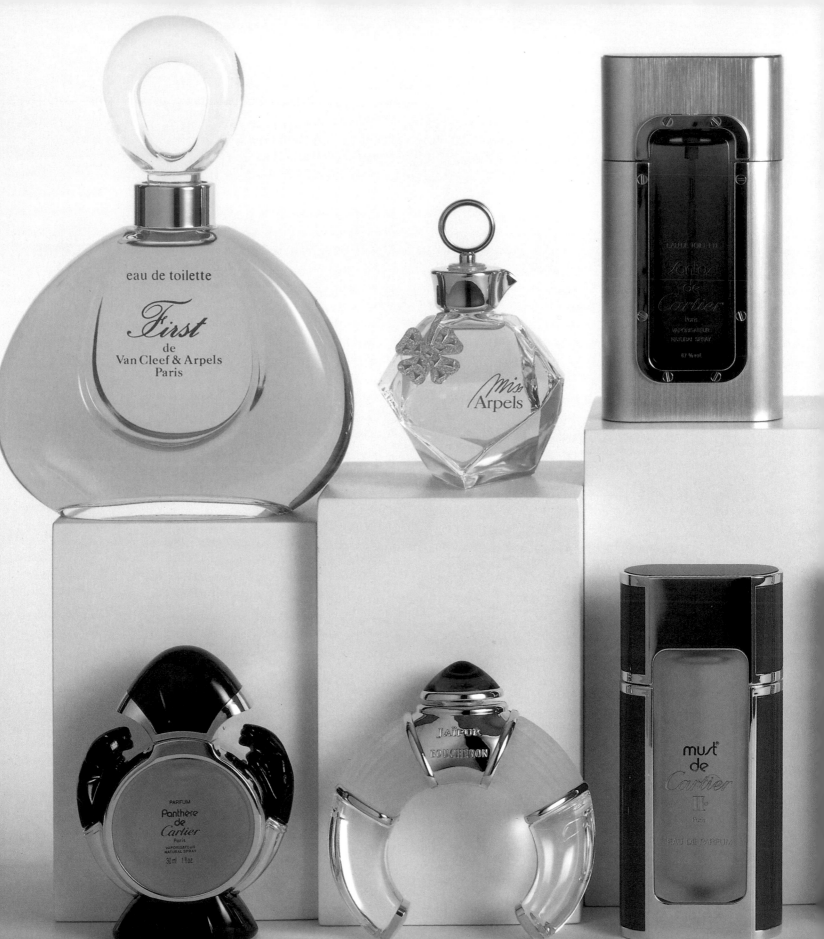

Top, left to right:
First *by Van Cleef & Arpels (eau de toilette) (1976).*
Miss Arpels *(1994).*
Santos *by Cartier (1981).*

Bottom, left to right:
Panthère *by Cartier (1987).*
Jaïpur *by Boucheron (1994).*
Must II *by Cartier (1993).*

This century has seen perfume secure a prized place in the luxury goods market. Jewelers have not been able to resist reflecting the fascinating world of metals and precious stones in a perfume bottle.

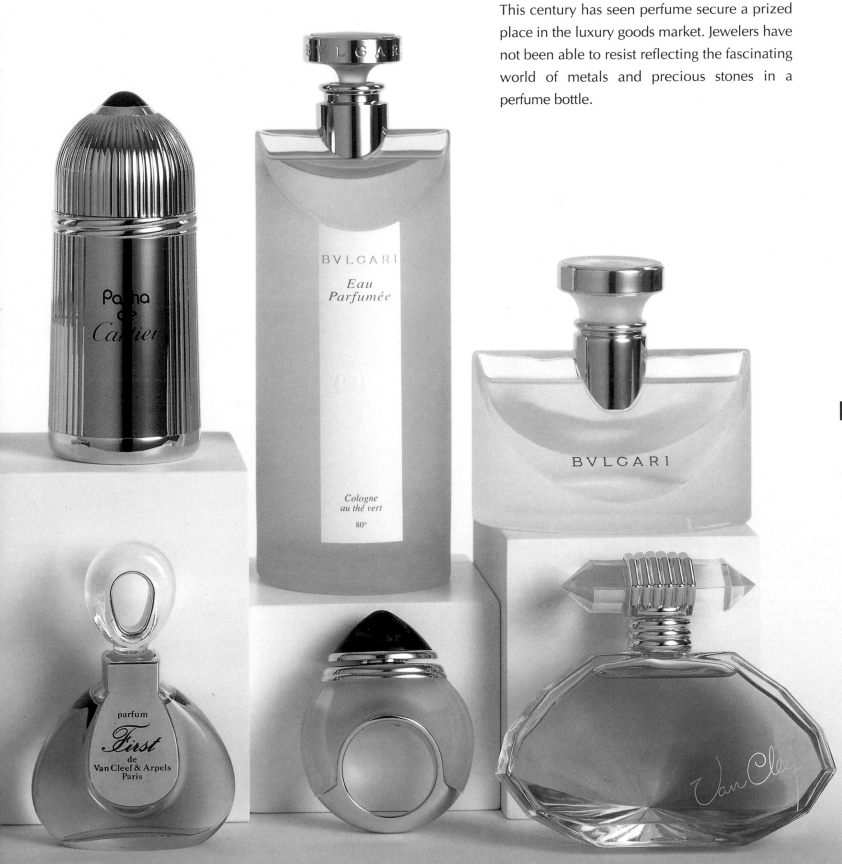

119

Top, left to right:
Pasha *by Cartier* (1992).
Eau Parfumée, Cologne au thé vert *by Bulgari* (1993).
Bulgari *(1994).*

Bottom, left to right:
First by *Van Cleef & Arpels (parfum)* (1976).
Boucheron *(1988).*
Van Cleef *(1993).*

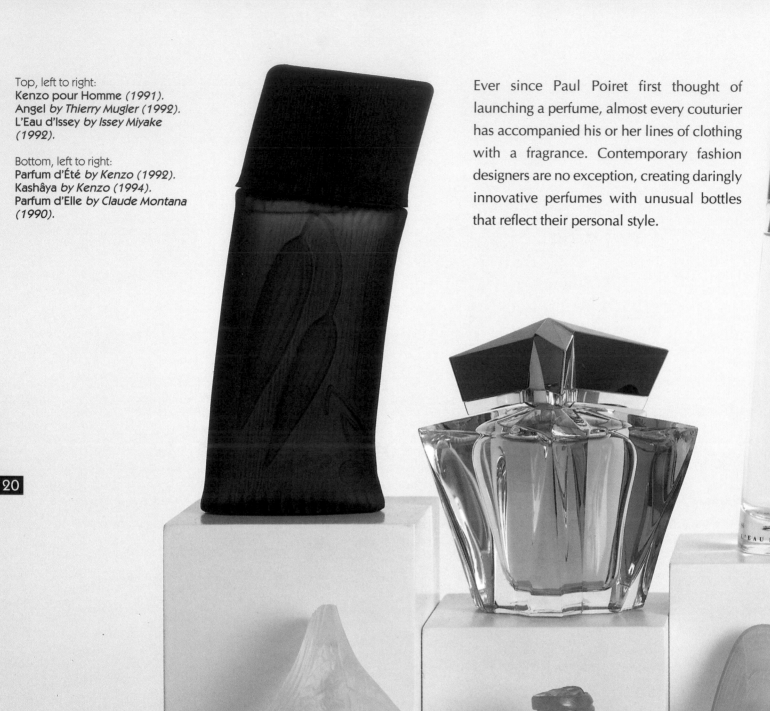

Top, left to right:
Kenzo pour Homme *(1991).*
Angel *by Thierry Mugler (1992).*
L'Eau d'Issey *by Issey Miyake (1992).*

Bottom, left to right:
Parfum d'Été *by Kenzo (1992).*
Kashâya *by Kenzo (1994).*
Parfum d'Elle *by Claude Montana (1990).*

Ever since Paul Poiret first thought of launching a perfume, almost every couturier has accompanied his or her lines of clothing with a fragrance. Contemporary fashion designers are no exception, creating daringly innovative perfumes with unusual bottles that reflect their personal style.

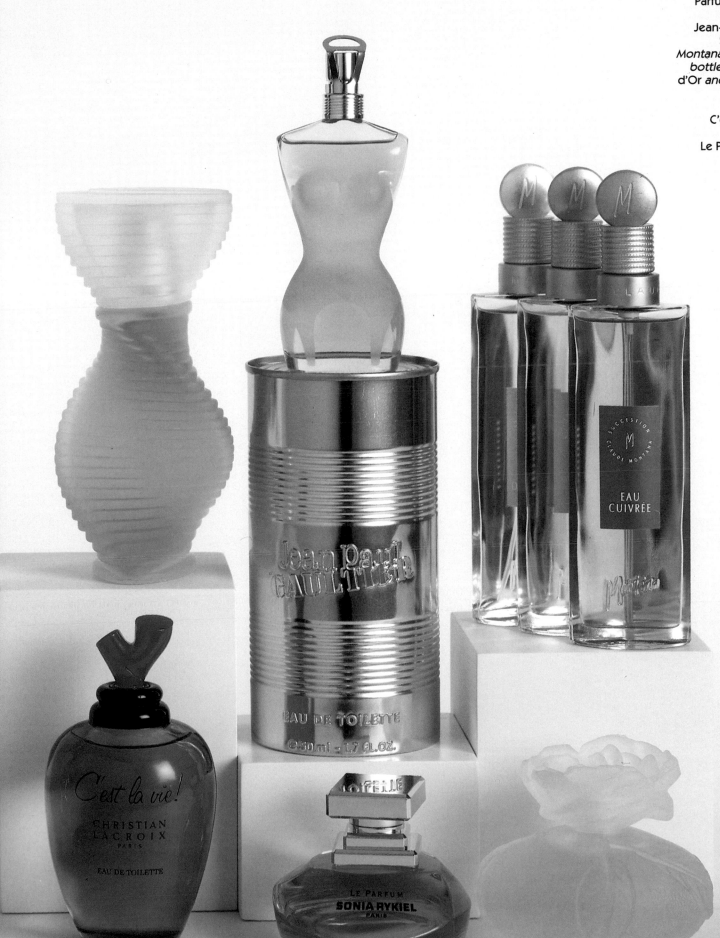

Top, left to right:
Parfum de Peau *by Claude Montana (1986).*
Jean-Paul Gaultier *(1993).*
Suggestion *by Claude Montana, with three different bottles –* Eau d'Argent, Eau d'Or *and* Eau Cuivrée *(1994).*

Bottom, left to right:
C'est la Vie! *by Christian Lacroix (1990).*
Le Parfum *by Sonia Rykiel (1993).*
Kenzo *(1988).*

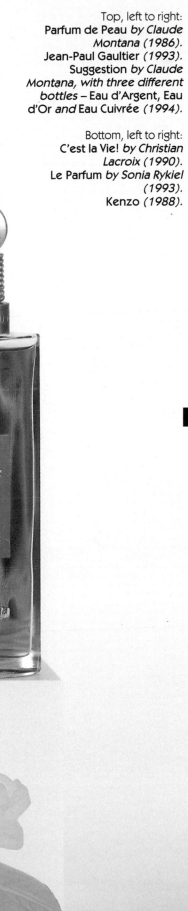

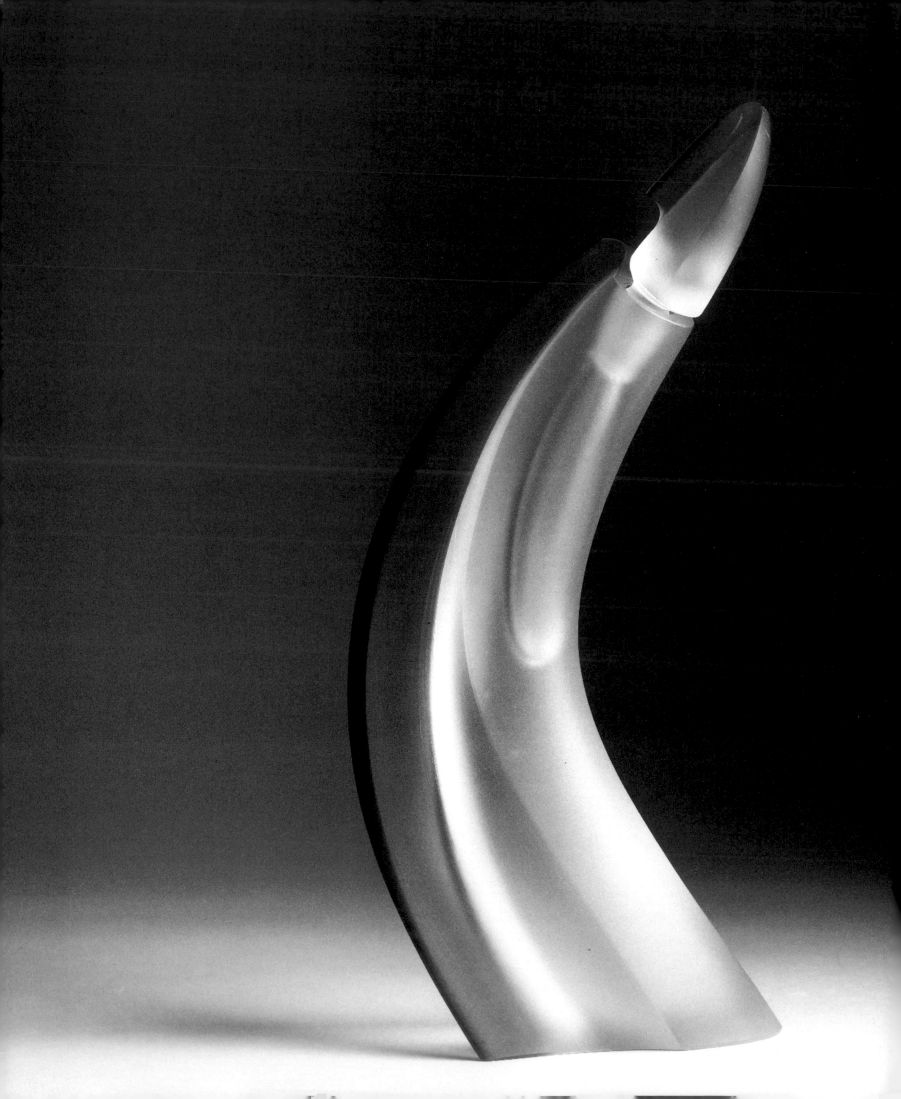

COLLECTIBLE BOTTLES

A few years ago, only a small number of connoisseurs collected perfume bottles. Today, however, these precious containers are extremely sought after and have become regular features at auction houses such as Drouot in Paris and Sotheby's in New York. The prices they fetch can be astronomical (often over 20,000 dollars), making them the preserve of a few wealthy (often American) collectors, or of major perfume-makers attempting to recover a part of their history. Once upon a time it was possible to find old bottles in bric-a-brac stores, but they have been all but plundered, as have most of our grandmothers' attics. Specialist shops dealing in just perfume bottles have since sprung up, and today there are a number of experts making a living in this field.

Bottles can be divided into two types: perfume containers, usually without a brand name and dating from Antiquity to the nineteenth century, which were sold empty and designed for a fragrance of the buyer's choice; and those which are specific to a particular fragrance, first appearing at the end of the last century, normally bearing the perfume-maker's name and containing one of his blends. Glass bottles are among the most desirable, while the plastic containers pioneered in the sixties are considered to be of little value. Lalique is undoubtedly one of the most sought after names, followed by Baccarat but also less famous names such as André Jollivet and Julien Viard. A bottle is judged according to its brand, date, originality of design and presence of the glass-maker's signature. Bottles made in the shape of animals, for example, are highly sought after, along with the baroque bottles of the eighteenth century or those which have a particular historical context. However, a bottle's value is determined mainly by its condition and presentation: a collectible bottle must have its original stopper and label, and is most valuable when still in its box. Bottles and packaging which have been restored are not at all valued by experts, nor are miniature samples, as numerous as their collectors may be. The bottles illustrated on the following pages all come from the DROM perfumery company's private collection, which was begun in the Twenties and now comprises 1,700 pieces all housed in a museum at Baierbrunn, near Munich in Germany.

Twentieth-century perfume bottle, DROM collection.

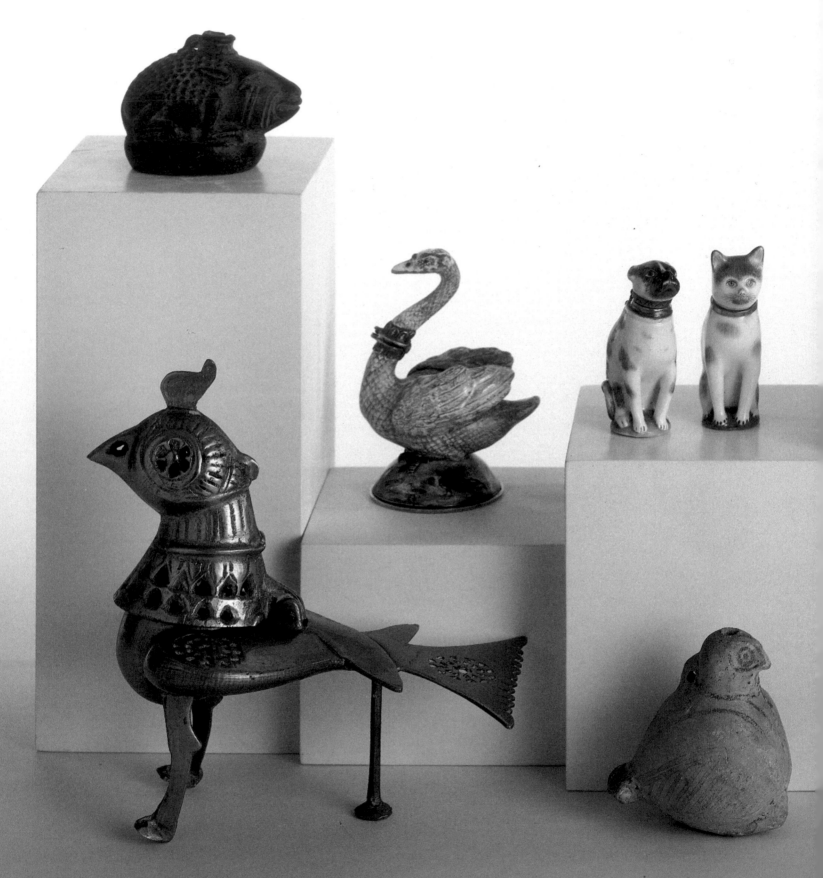

Top, left to right:
Black clay ointment pot in the shape of a porcupine, Roman-Ptolemaic Egypt (possibly Syrian-influenced), 3rd-1st century BC.
Silver and enamel bottle in the shape of a swan, Vienna, Austria, late 19th century.
Painted porcelain bottle in the shape of a pug dog, with silver fittings, Germany (probably Meissen), 18th century.
Painted porcelain bottle in the shape of a cat, Germany (possibly Thuringe), 18th-19th century.

Bottom, left to right:
Brass perfume-burner in the shape of a bird with hinged, openworked head to allow the perfume to escape, India, 20th century.
Corinthian, pale-colored and painted clay holy oil jar in the shape of a nesting owl, 6th century BC.

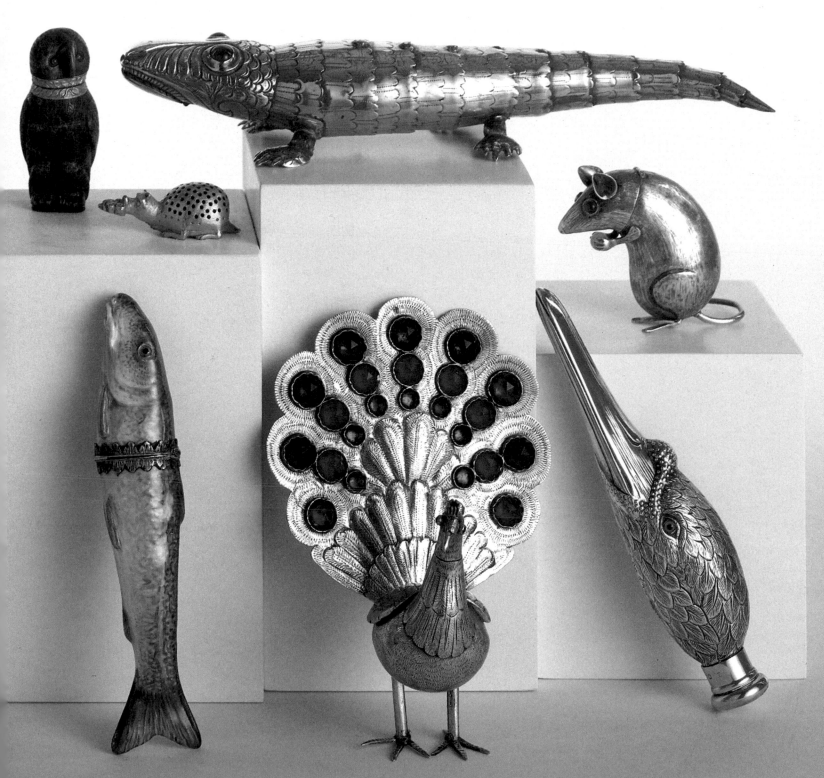

Top, left to right:
Labradorite bottle in the shape of an owl, with eyes made of rubies and a gold collar, Germany, c.1810.
Gilded bronze pomander in the shape of a hippopotamus, Iran, 20th century.
Engraved silver scent box in the shape of a crocodile, with articulated joints and eyes made of red garnet, probably Mexican, 19th century.
Silver scent box in the shape of a mouse, bearing the mark of master silversmith Christian Raphael Schmidt, Denmark, early 19th century.

Bottom, left to right:
Painted porcelain scent box in the shape of a fish, with silver mount, Germany (possibly Thuringe), 18th century.
Silver scent box in the shape of a peacock, bearing the mark of Christian Raphael Schmidt (1753-1822), with articulated wings and a removable head, its eyes and feathers decorated with colored glass. Denmark, early 19th century.
Silver handbag bottle in the shape of a bird's head, S. Mordan & Co. England, 1886.

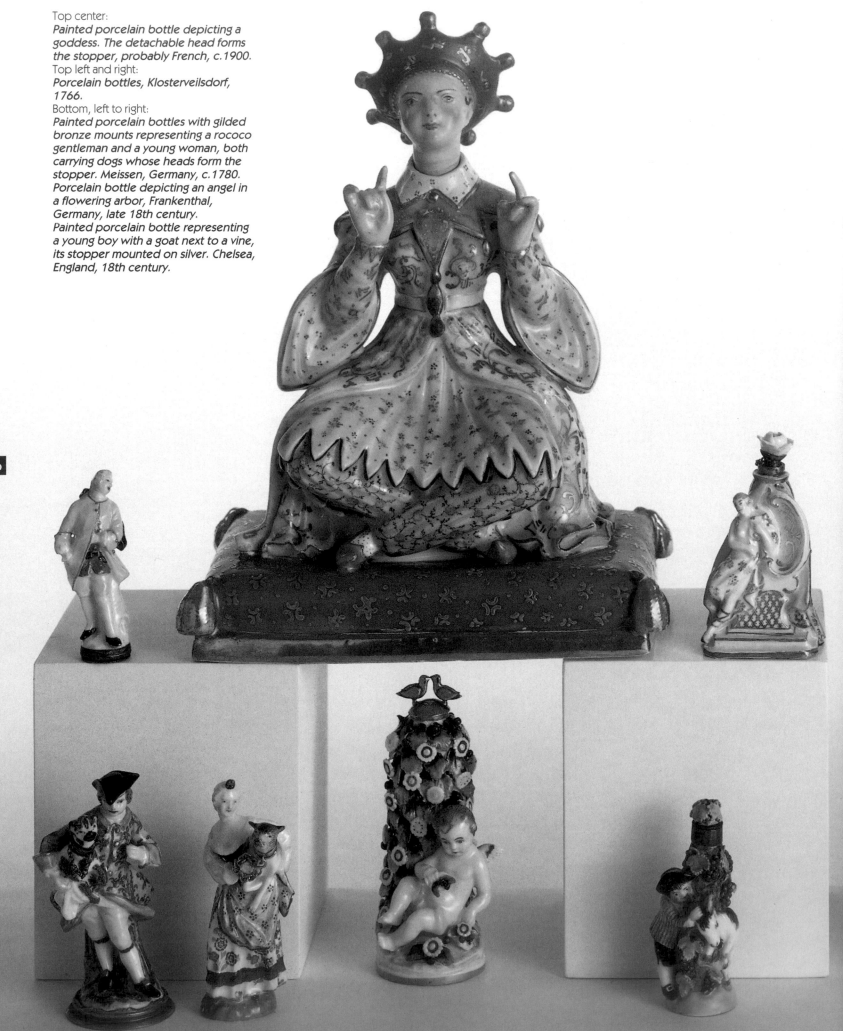

Top center:
Painted porcelain bottle depicting a goddess. The detachable head forms the stopper, probably French, c.1900.
Top left and right:
Porcelain bottles, Klosterveilsdorf, 1766.
Bottom, left to right:
Painted porcelain bottles with gilded bronze mounts representing a rococo gentleman and a young woman, both carrying dogs whose heads form the stopper. Meissen, Germany, c.1780. Porcelain bottle depicting an angel in a flowering arbor, Frankenthal, Germany, late 18th century. Painted porcelain bottle representing a young boy with a goat next to a vine, its stopper mounted on silver. Chelsea, England, 18th century.

126

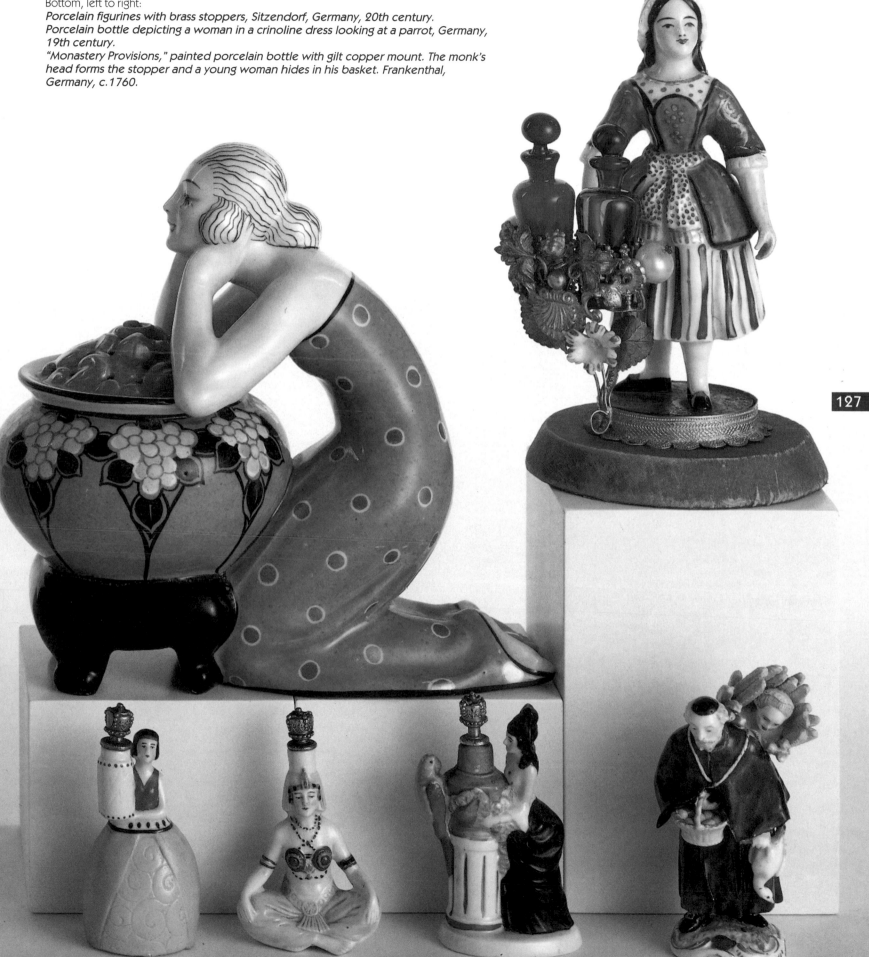

Top, left to right:
Porcelain pot-pourri jar, France, 1920-1930.
Porcelain figure of a young girl with a basket containing two small glass and metal bottles, probably French, 19th or 20th century.
Bottom, left to right:
Porcelain figurines with brass stoppers, Sitzendorf, Germany, 20th century.
Porcelain bottle depicting a woman in a crinoline dress looking at a parrot, Germany, 19th century.
"Monastery Provisions," painted porcelain bottle with gilt copper mount. The monk's head forms the stopper and a young woman hides in his basket. Frankenthal, Germany, c.1760.

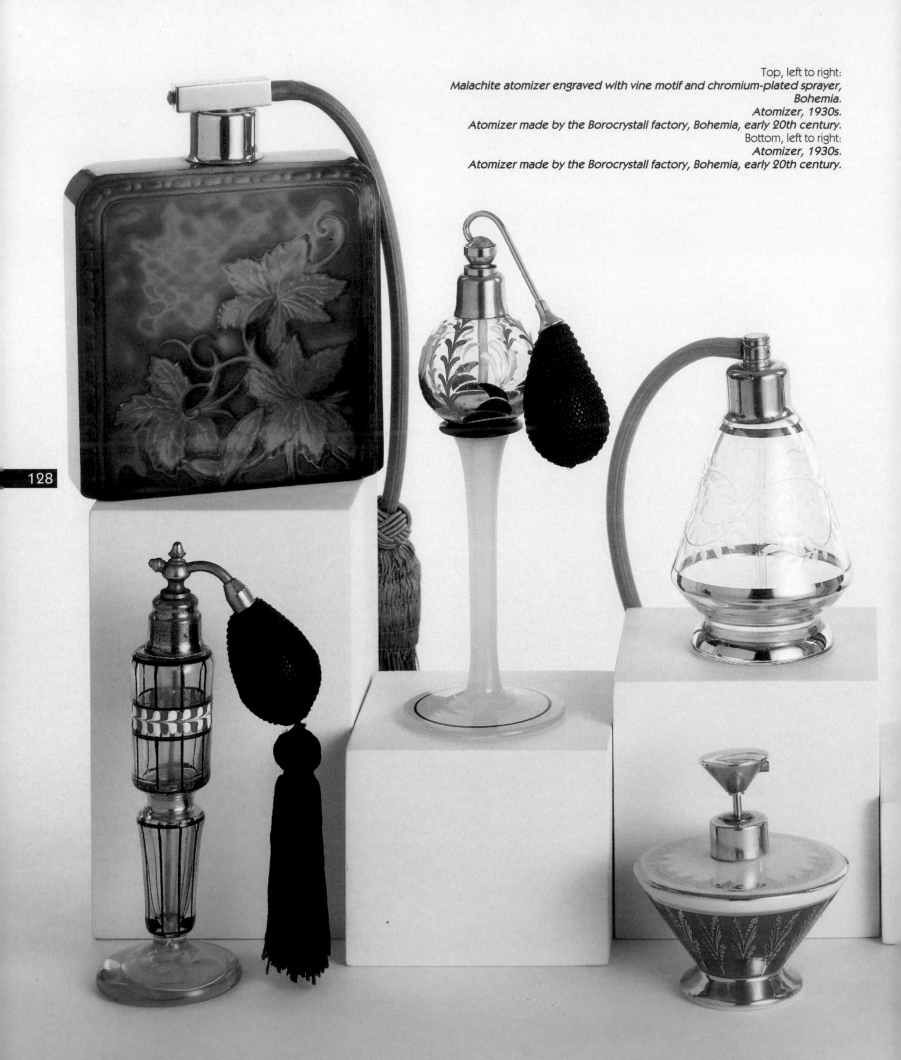

Top, left to right:
Malachite atomizer engraved with vine motif and chromium-plated sprayer, Bohemia.
Atomizer, 1930s.
Atomizer made by the Borocrystall factory, Bohemia, early 20th century.
Bottom, left to right:
Atomizer, 1930s.
Atomizer made by the Borocrystall factory, Bohemia, early 20th century.

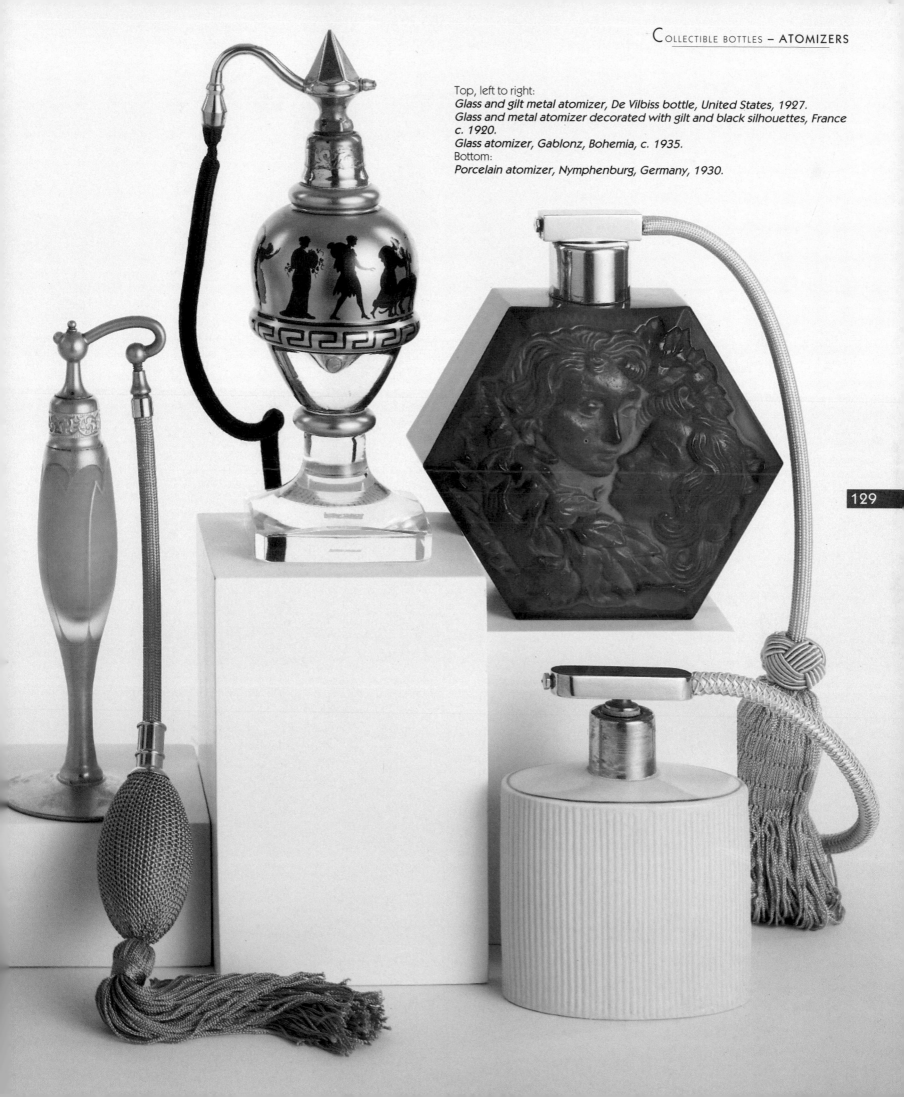

Top, left to right:
Glass and gilt metal atomizer, De Vilbiss bottle, United States, 1927.
Glass and metal atomizer decorated with gilt and black silhouettes, France c. 1920.
Glass atomizer, Gablonz, Bohemia, c. 1935.
Bottom:
Porcelain atomizer, Nymphenburg, Germany, 1930.

Top, left to right:
Tiffany glass and copper gilt bottle, signed LCTO, early 20th century.
Art Nouveau yellow glass bottle with wine-colored orchid decoration and gilded atomizer, created by Émile Gallé.
Conical bottle in "verre de soie" (a technique introduced in 1905), designed by Frederick Carder, United States, c.1905.
Bottom, left to right:
Pear-shaped perfume-burner with cyclamen design, Argental glass works, France, c.1910.
Bottle in nephrite (a type of jade), silver, diamonds and pearls, with moiré enamel decorated with guilloches, bearing the mark of Henrick Wigström, St Petersburg, Russia, early 20th century.
Glass and silver perfume-burner with leaf and flower motifs, created by Émile Gallé, Nancy, France, c.1905.

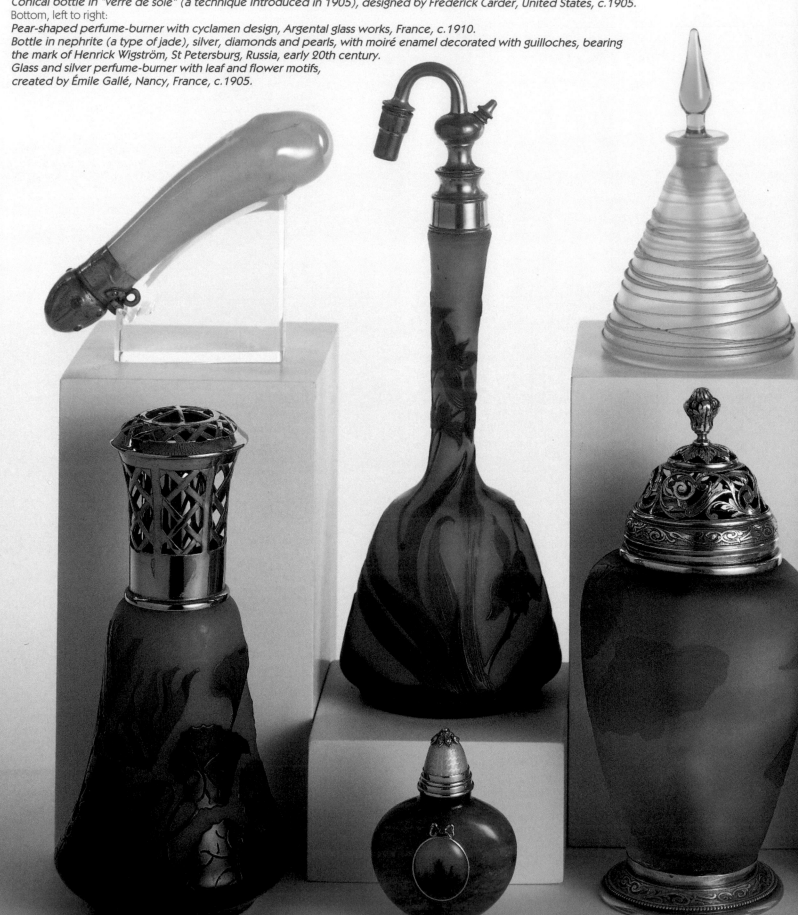

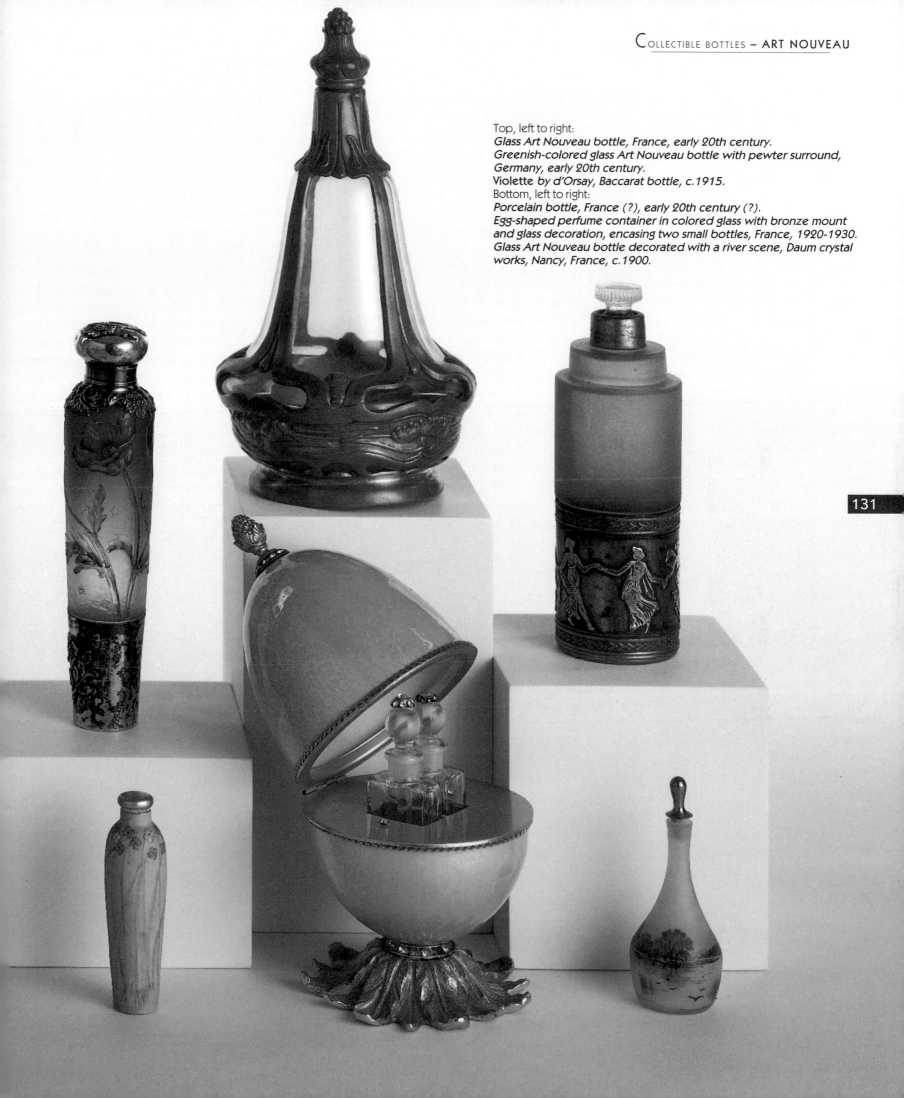

Top, left to right:
Glass Art Nouveau bottle, France, early 20th century.
Greenish-colored glass Art Nouveau bottle with pewter surround, Germany, early 20th century.
Violette by d'Orsay, Baccarat bottle, c.1915.
Bottom, left to right:
Porcelain bottle, France (?), early 20th century (?).
Egg-shaped perfume container in colored glass with bronze mount and glass decoration, encasing two small bottles, France, 1920-1930.
Glass Art Nouveau bottle decorated with a river scene, Daum crystal works, Nancy, France, c.1900.

Glass and copper bottle,
Bohemia or Venice, 19th century.

Enamel and silver
perfume baton,
England, 20th century.

Bottle for rose oil,
Bohemia, 1825.

Crystal and silver-plated brass
bottle, Bohemia, 20th century.

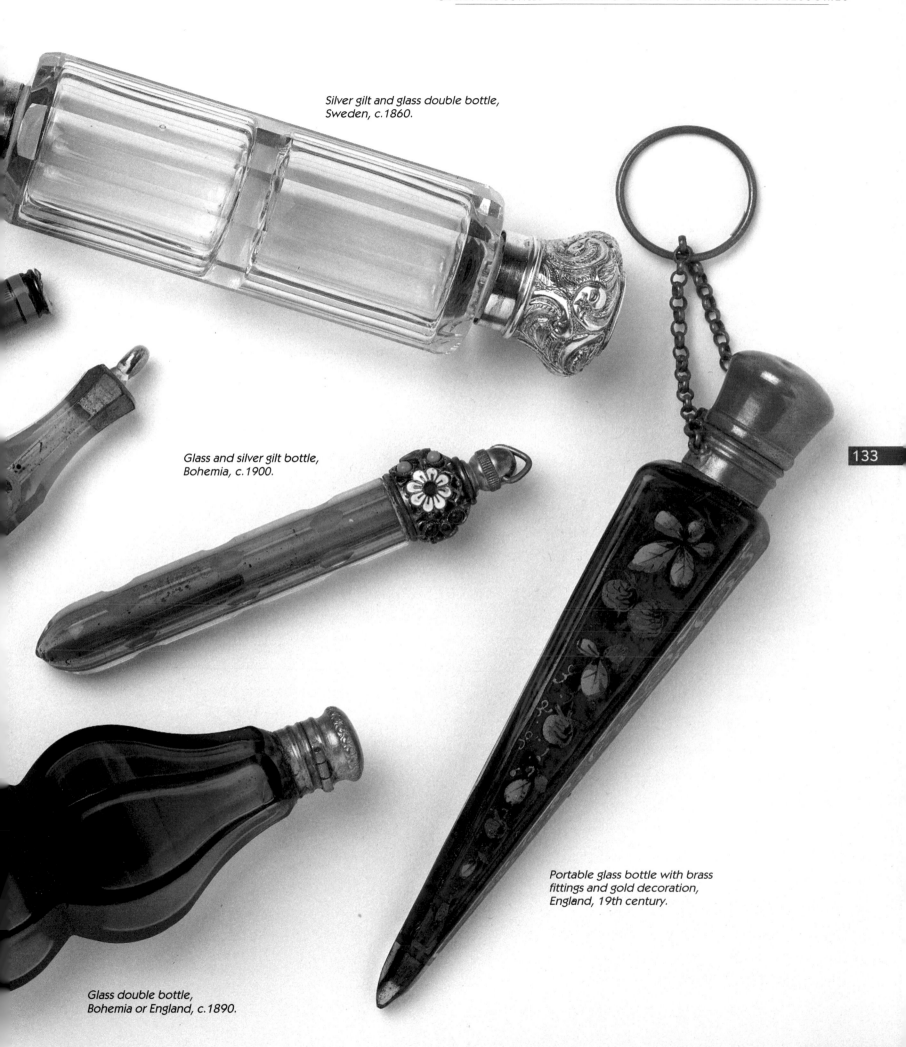

Silver gilt and glass double bottle,
Sweden, c.1860.

Glass and silver gilt bottle,
Bohemia, c.1900.

Portable glass bottle with brass
fittings and gold decoration,
England, 19th century.

Glass double bottle,
Bohemia or England, c.1890.

Vinaigrette bracelet
containing a lock of hair, Italy,
late 19th century.

Glass bottle with brass fittings,
Bohemia, 20th century.

Silver bottle,
Hungary, 20th century.

Glass bottle with brass fittings,
Belgium, c.1920.

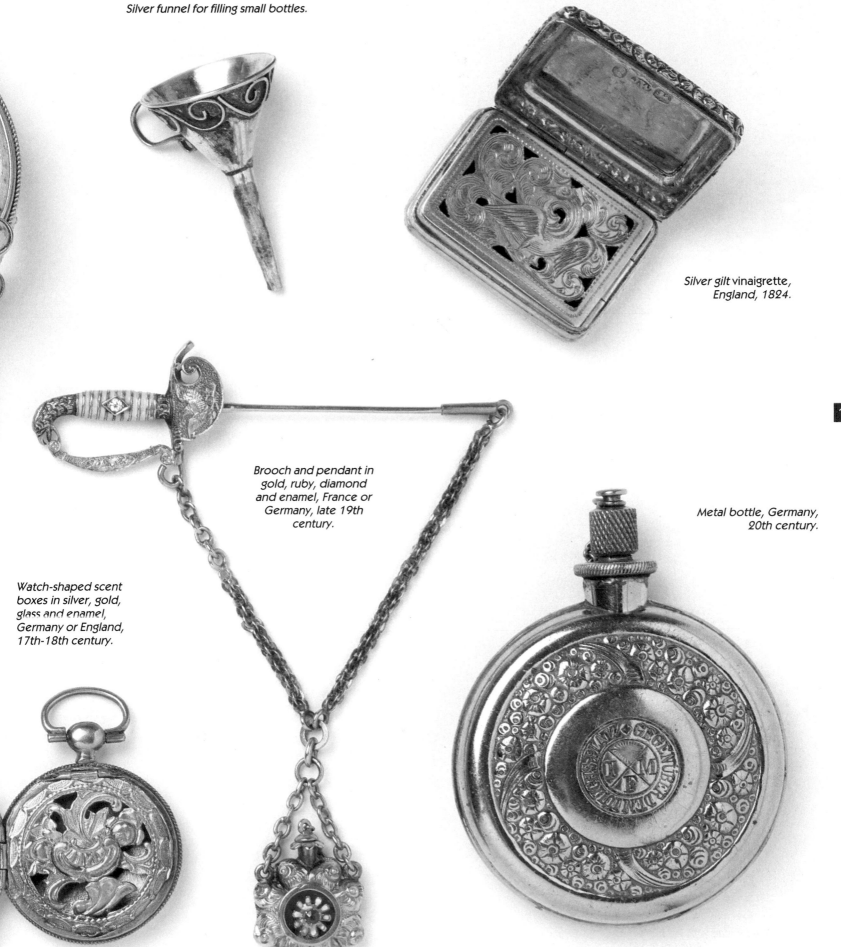

Silver funnel for filling small bottles.

Silver gilt vinaigrette, England, 1824.

Brooch and pendant in gold, ruby, diamond and enamel, France or Germany, late 19th century.

Metal bottle, Germany, 20th century.

Watch-shaped scent boxes in silver, gold, glass and enamel, Germany or England, 17th-18th century.

CRYSTAL AND GLASS MAKERS

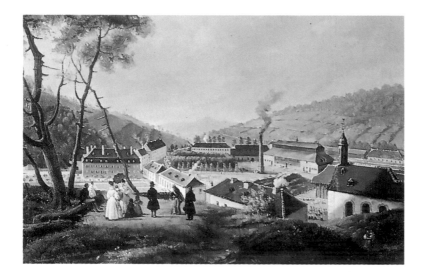

A craftsman at the Saint-Louis crystal factory. Making a crystal bottle demands great manual skill.

The royal Saint-Louis glass-works was established in 1767 in Lorraine.

After manufacture, glass is engraved on a wheel.

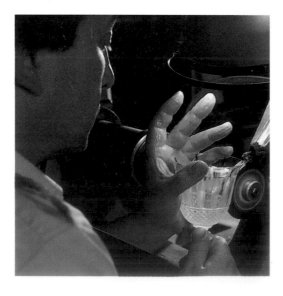

A supremely neutral material, whose transparency borders on intangibility, glass was destined to contain dreams. Where they could afford to, the Romans kept their precious, fragrant ointments in containers made from murra (an iridescent substance similar to glass) or engraved or blown glass, rather than terracotta pots. The technique of glass-blowing, developed along the Syrian coast just before the birth of Christ, led to a proliferation of containers in countless new shapes – phials and ampullae for perfume, jars for balsam and so on. After the fall of the Roman Empire, however, both the practice of using perfumes and the advanced art of glass-making slipped into obscurity. It was not until the thirteenth century that Venice established its first glass-works on the island of Murano, which rapidly gained a high reputation all over Europe. The secret of the Venetian craftsmen lay in the use of seaweed ashes to create sodium glass. However, Venetian superiority was to be overturned in the seventeenth century by the development of crystal in England and Bohemia. The addition of lead, in England, or potash, in Bohemia, produced a heavier and more transparent material than ordinary glass, qualities which made it better suited to engraving on a wheel. In 1736, possibly with the help of immigrant Bohemian craftsmen, a Venetian named Giuseppe Briati in turn mastered the art of crystal-making, and production of engraved glass began in the city. This came too late, however, to halt the decline of the Murano glass-works. From the mid-seventeenth century onwards, the city of Modena enjoyed similar fame for its more utilitarian output, which consisted mainly of tableware and window glass.

In France, a charter drawn up in 1448 granted official recognition to "gentlemen glass-makers" and forbade commoners from practicing the art. Notable developments in the industry then took place in France, where the Duke of Anjou had lured glass-makers from Murano and Bohemia. With its sandstone, salt-works and potash derived from bracken ashes, the region of Lorraine proved an ideal location. The processes involved in the manufacture of this mysterious material were shrouded in the utmost secrecy and the local glass-makers swore an oath never to reveal their craft to anyone but their male offspring.

Government protectionism limiting imports of glass from Bohemia and England led to the establishment of two of the most famous glass-works in France: production of window glass and Bohemian-style tableware began in the village of Baccarat, on the banks of the River Meurthe, in 1765; in 1767, about sixty miles to the north at Saint-Louis-lès-Bitche, the Saint-Louis royal glass-works opened. The formula for making lead crystal, identical to English flint glass, was brought to France in 1781 by its director. The stakes involved were so high that in order to protect the secret, the state banned employees from moving more than three miles away from the factory and demanded that they give two years' notice before leaving the company. However, as a result of the French Revolution, luxury industries fared badly in the next few years. Although Saint-Louis managed to maintain production and then expand from 1800 onwards, the Baccarat glass-works struggled to survive until 1816, when it was bought and elevated to the rank of crystal manufacturer by a former director at Saint-Louis. The victorious middle classes made crystal a symbol of their rise to prominence. Evidence of this can be seen in the sumptuous tableware, glittering chandeliers and elaborate perfume bottles of the period.

The manufacture of perfume bottles began in earnest at Saint-Louis in the 1830s, with the invention of molding which meant that glass-makers could reproduce the famous "diamond cut." After the development of filigree work in 1837 and of the use of color in 1844, opaline crystal was introduced. The most exceptional bottles were created between 1848 and 1850. Glass-makers at the time could work from an extensive palette and apply layers of different colored opaline to create an infinite variety of iridescent effects. Flat-sided cut glass pieces began to appear and, sometime around the 1870s, acid engraving made possible the gold decoration which became a Saint-Louis speciality. From 1925 onwards, Saint-Louis produced bottles for the major perfume-makers of the time such as François Coty, L.T. Piver, Bourjois and Jean Patou. The manufacturer also distinguished itself with the creation of the famous square bottle for Chanel No.5 and its work for Dior and Balmain after the Second World War.

The Baccarat crystal-works followed a similar course, building a new glass-cutting section in 1907 to respond to Increasing demand from the burgeoning perfumery industry. Four years later, the raising of production levels to five thousand bottles per day necessitated a further extension. The order book contains all the major names in perfumery: Coty, Houbigant, and Guerlain, for whose *Mitsouko* and *L'Heure Bleue* Baccarat designed a remarkable stopper shaped like a gendarme's hat. After the First World War, Baccarat created bottles for Paul Poiret, Jean Patou and Elizabeth Arden, including the hand for *It's You*. In 1945, the workshops produced Dali's design for *Le Roy Soleil* then, later, bottles for numerous Dior creations and, more recently, for Paco Rabanne and Versace. Developments at Lalique, in the meantime, included a process by which elaborate pieces of crystal could be made by machine. René Lalique went on to create bottles that contributed in large measure to the success of perfumes by Coty, Roger & Gallet, Houbigant, d'Orsay, Worth and the majority of well-known perfume-makers. After the Second World War, his son Marc worked mainly for Nina Ricci and is responsible for the timeless grace of the entwined doves of *L'Air du Temps*.

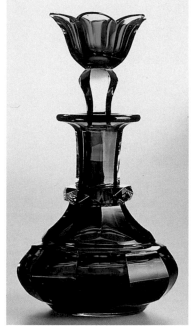
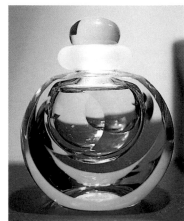

Two bottles produced by the Saint-Louis crystal factory:
Left: *A design from around 1850.*
Below: L'Eau de Saint-Louis *(1992).*

137

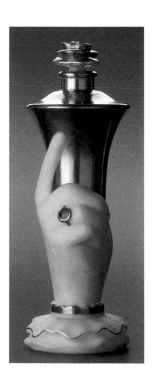

Cyclamen *by Elizabeth Arden. Created in 1939 in Baccarat milk glass, the bottle is in the shape of an opened fan topped by a tall, conical, transparent crystal stopper.*

It's You *by Elizabeth Arden. This bottle, made in 1939, is one of the Baccarat crystal factory's most famous creations.*

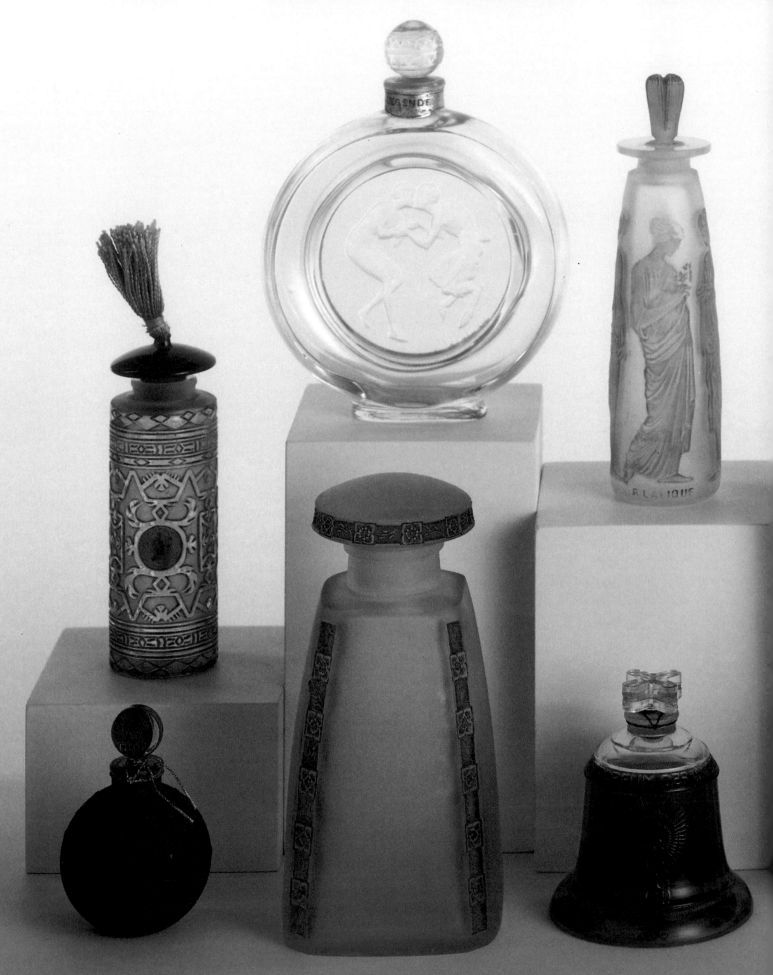

138

Top, left to right:
Les Parfums de Rosine *by Paul Poiret, Murano glass bottle, Paris,*
1925.
Lalique bottle.
Ambre Antique *by Coty, Lalique bottle, 1907.*

Bottom, left to right:
Dans la Nuit *by Worth, Lalique bottle.*
Lalique's "Fleurette" design, c.1930.
Le Parfum des Anges, *created to mark the opening of the Oviatt*
building in Los Angeles, Lalique bottle, 1928.

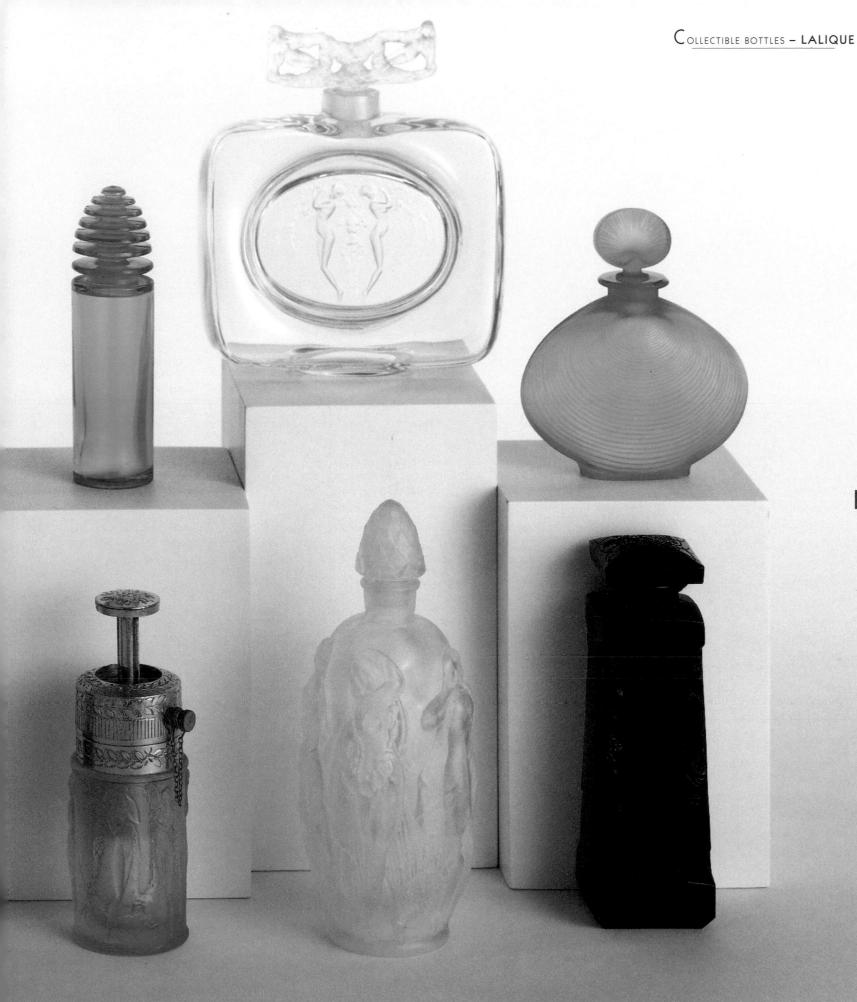

Top, left to right:
Sans Adieu by Worth, Lalique bottle, 1929.
A relief of two figures designed by Lalique, 1912.
Lalique's "La Telline" design in green glass, 1920.

Bottom, left to right:
Glass and gilt bronze atomizer, Lalique bottle.
Lalique bottle.
Ambre d'Orsay, Lalique bottle , 1920-1930.

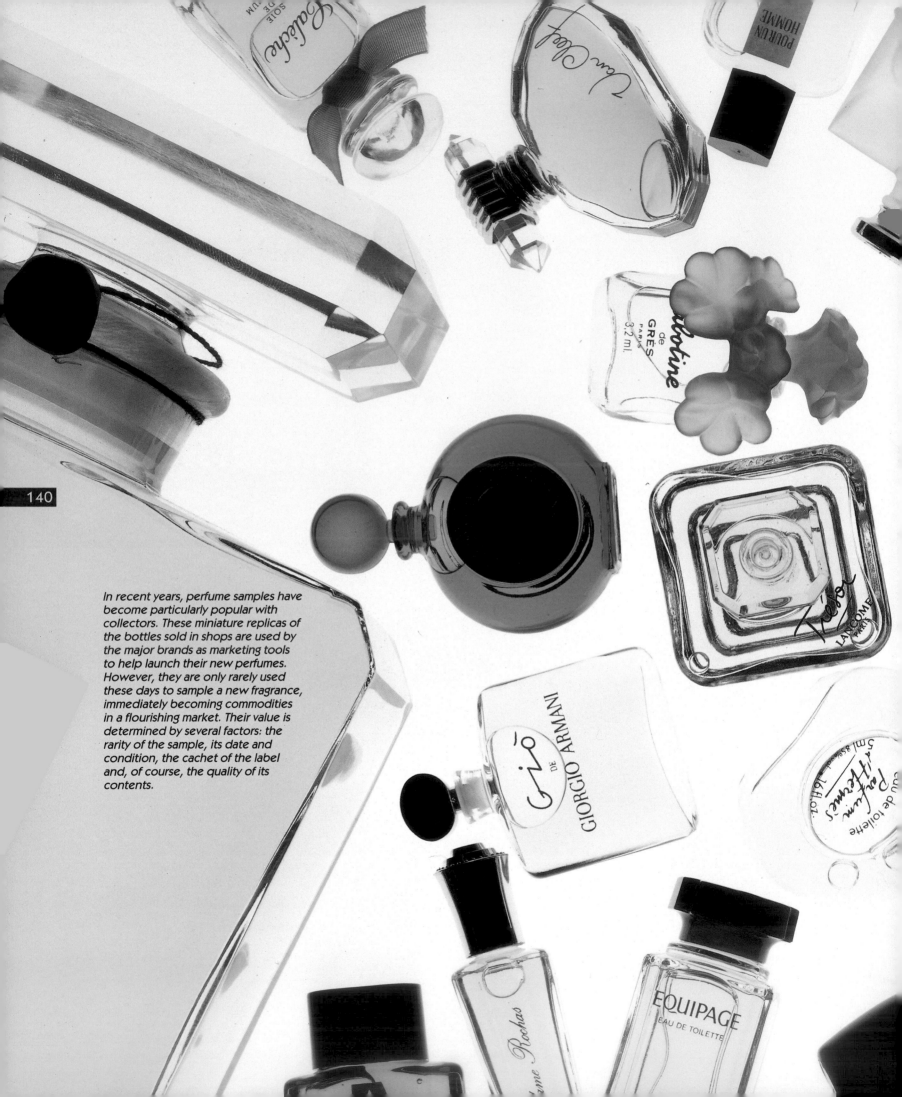

In recent years, perfume samples have become particularly popular with collectors. These miniature replicas of the bottles sold in shops are used by the major brands as marketing tools to help launch their new perfumes. However, they are only rarely used these days to sample a new fragrance, immediately becoming commodities in a flourishing market. Their value is determined by several factors: the rarity of the sample, its date and condition, the cachet of the label and, of course, the quality of its contents.

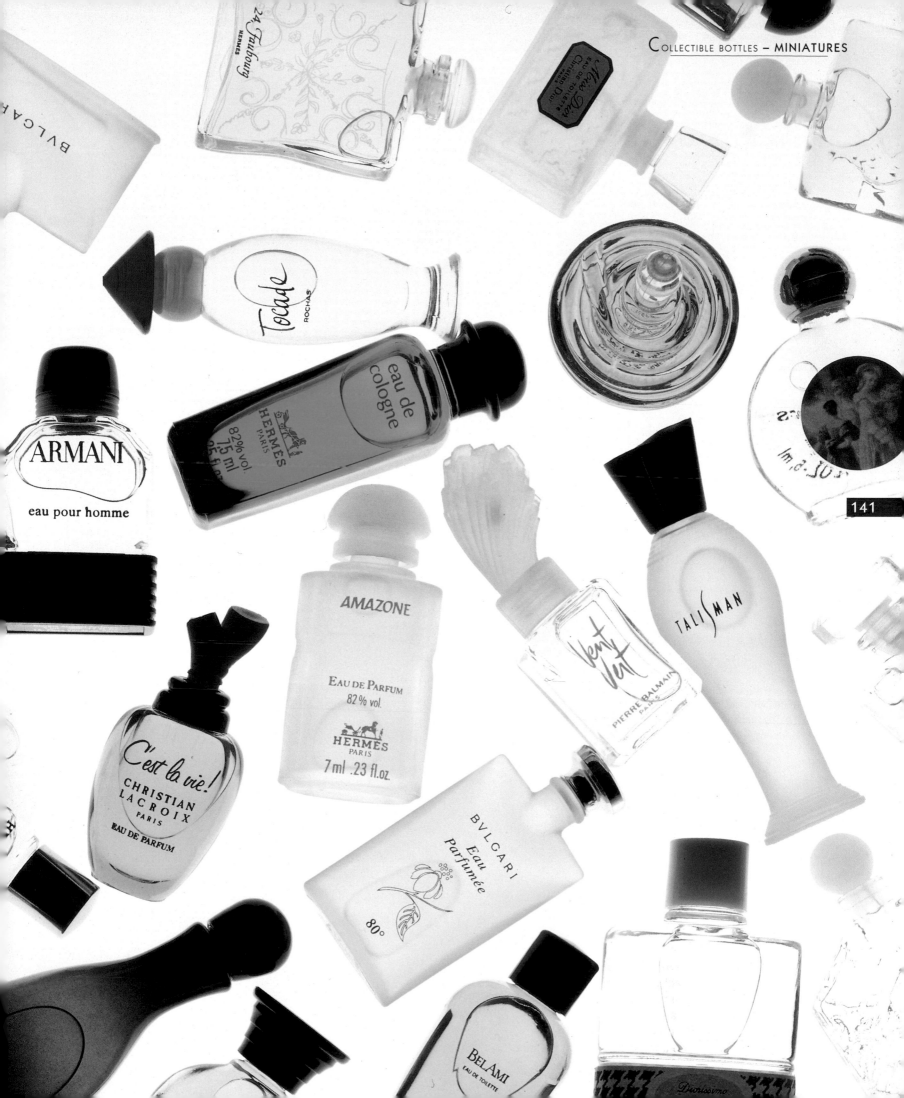

141

ACKNOWLEDGEMENTS

The author would like to thank the many people who have helped her produce this book and who, with their co-operation and invaluable knowledge, enabled her to explore "the world of perfume."

Thanks especially to:
Bruno Storp, managing director of the DROM perfumery company, Baierbrunn, Germany; Ursula Storp, curator of the DROM perfume bottle collection, who allowed us to take photographs, and Sylvia Dubois; Karine Dubreuil, chief perfume-blender at DROM, for her friendly patience and clear explanations; Michel Maunier-Rossi, head of DROM France; Danièle Michelet, Laurence Balland and Laurence Renaud at the *Fédération des industries de la parfumerie*; Marie-Hélène Gourmelon at the *Comité français du partum*; the technical department of the *Société française des parfumeurs* and Jean Kerléo, for his insightful interview; the perfume-blenders Françoise Caron, Éric Houdou and Olivier Cresp; perfume-blender Jacques Polge, Nathalie Franchini and Laetitia Colas at Chanel; Éliane de la Béraudière at Christian Dior; Élisabeth Sirot and Emily Jeangeorges at Guerlain; Maddy Nicot at Hermès; Monique Sarris and Blandine Viry at Lancôme; Odile Fraigneau at Lanvin; managing director Jean de Moüy, perfume-blender Jean Kerléo and Valérie Dufournier at Jean Patou; Ève Leporq and Michèle Tibout at Nina Ricci; Danièle Paquier at Rochas; Caroline Régin and Jean Davy at Roger & Gallet; Monique Gossart at Yardley; research director Jacques-Marie Decazes and François Huyghes-Despointes at Givaudan Roure; Frédérique von Eben-Worlée at the Monique Rémy Laboratory for her assistance with pictures; Fabienne de Sèze at Baccarat; Martine Oswald and Andréa Buchin at Saint-Louis; Colette Tronel at the Fragonard Perfume Museum, for her assistance with pictures; Marika Genty at Dior Couture, for her assistance with pictures; Jeannine Mongin for her knowledge and assistance with pictures; Tracey Glowinski at Firmenich, for her assistance with pictures; Xavier Dujoncquoy at Muelhens.

Thanks also to all the press offices who kindly lent their bottles to be photographed.

PHOTOGRAPHIC CREDITS

BIBLIOGRAPHY

J.Alaux, F.Bajot, S.de Chirée, P.Mauriès,
Lanvin
Ricci, 1988

Baccarat, les flacons à parfum,
Compagnie des cristalliers de Baccarat, Éditions H.Addor, 1994

Jacqueline Blanc-Mouchet
Odeurs
Autrement, 1987

Jean-François Blayn (ed.)
Question de parfumerie,
essai sur l'art et la creation en parfumerie
Éditions Corpman, 1988

Monique Cabré,
Échantillons de parfums,
Syros Alternatives, 1991

Carla Cerutti,
Flacons,
Celiv, 1994

Edmonde Charles-Roux,
Le Temps Chanel,
Chêne-Grasset, 1979

Maurice Chastrette,
L'Art des parfums,
Hachette,1995

Comité Français des Parfums,
Classification des parfums, 1990

Alain Corbin,
Le Miasme et la Jonquille,
Aubier, 1982

Jacqueline Demornex,
Lancôme,
Éditions du Regard, 1985

Pierre Dinand,
Les formes du parfum, trente ans de design,
Belfond, 1990

Meredith Etherington-Smith
Patou,
Denoël, 1984

Joseph Farnarier,
Contribution à la connaissance de la ville de Grasse,
Parfumerie, 1983

Colette Fellous,
Guerlain,
Denoël, 1987

Geneviève Fontan and Nathalie Barnouin,
Parfums d'exception,
Milan, 1993

Sylvie Girard,
Le Livre du parfum,
Messidor, 1990

Françoise Giroud,
Christian Dior,
Éditions du Regard, 1987

Hymne au parfum,
Catalogue from the exhibition at the
Musée des Arts et de la Mode, 1990-1991

Gérard Ingold,
Saint-Louis, de l'art du verre à l'art du cristal,
de 1586 à nos jours,
Denoël, 1986

Serge Manseau,
Les Flacons,
La Martinière, 1995

Maurice Maurin and Jean-François Blayn,
Dictionnaire du langage parfumé,
Éditions Quarante Huit Publicité, 1993

Christine Mayer-Lefkowith,
L'Art du parfum,
Celiv, 1994

Paul Morand,
L'Allure de Chanel,
Hermann, 1976

Les Nouvelles de l'Osmothèque,
Periodic newsletter published by the
Versailles osmothèque.

Ghislaine Pillivuyt,
Histoire du parfum,
Denoël, 1988

Marie-France Pochna,
Christian Dior,
Flammarion, 1994

Marie-France Pochna,
Nina Ricci,
Éditions du Regard, 1992

Eugène Rimmel,
Le Livre des parfums,
Les Éditions 1900, 1990

Edmond Roudnitska,
Le Parfum,
Que sais-je? P.U.F., 1994

Edmond Roudnitska,
Sous le signe du parfum,
Éditions de l'Albaron, Société Présence du livre, 1991

Maïté Turonnet,
Parlons parfum,
Mondo, 1993

J.Winand, M.Malaise, C.Fontinoy, M.Meyskens,
R.Laruelle, J.Hadorn,
L'Art du parfum,
Le Temps apprivoisé, 1993